THE UNTOLD STORY OF KIM

"A true story of one
woman's triumph
over pain."

THE UNTOLD
STORY OF KIM

Ed Robinson

"Natural forces in us are the true healers of disease."

—Hippocrates

This book is dedicated first to my wife, the lovely Miss Kim. Its purpose is to provide hope for the many thousands who suffer from chronic pain and to raise the awareness of poorly understood pain syndromes such as RSD/CRPS.

TABLE OF CONTENTS

PRELUDE

I CAME HOME FROM WORK TO find Kim lying on the living room floor. She was curled up in the fetal position clutching her affected leg with both arms. She was crying. I'm not talking about a whimper. I'm talking about a full blown sobbing wail.

I dropped whatever I was carrying and rushed to her side. I held her head in my lap and stroked her hair, not knowing what else to do. She looked up at me through tear soaked eyes and said, "Cut my leg off. Please, make it go away."

This is life with RSD.

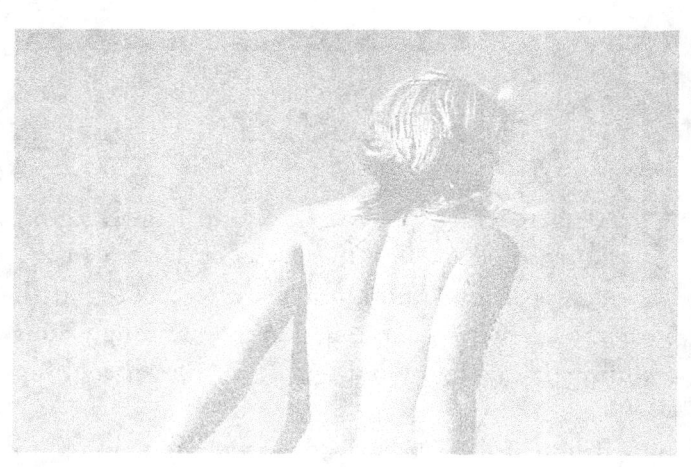

IT'S JOE BIDEN'S FAULT!

K IM'S POSITION AT DOVER DOWNS Hotel and Casino was as a banquet captain. She was very proud of her achievements and worked hard to be a success. Throughout her time there she got to meet many celebrities, singing acts and NASCAR drivers. She particularly enjoyed taking care of famous country singers like Jason Aldean and Jake Owen.

On this day she was to host a fundraiser for Vice Presidential candidate Joe Biden. It was October 14, 2008, just weeks away from the presidential election. She arrived at work to find Biden's security team forbidding entrance to all employees. Each one would have to wait their turn, eventually being subjected to an invasive pat down, security questionnaire and metal detection. A long line formed while tall men in dark suits decided if anyone was a threat.

Entering the building woefully behind schedule, employees rushed to catch up. Nervous about botching the most important event of her career, Kim came to the aid of her employees and began to set tables and make coffee. Even her boss was enlisted in the effort. All normal sense of routine was lost. Servers ran about in all directions and caution was thrown to the wind.

As Kim crouched down to retrieve an extra coffee urn from a low shelf, her boss was running down the hall pushing a speed cart. This is a large metal device designed to carry dozens of food trays at once. In his haste he never saw her. The heavy metal cart threw Kim across the hall. The point of impact was at the base of her spine, slightly into her left buttock.

It was a day she would never forget. It was also the last day she would ever work at Dover Downs.

At the hospital it was thought she may have broken her tailbone. X-rays however, were negative. An MRI discovered a torn hamstring, and damage to something called the piriformis muscle, which runs along the sciatic nerve through the buttock and into the upper thigh.

She was referred to an orthopedic surgeon whom I'll call Christian doctor. He was a very nice man who wore a large gold cross around his neck. He seemed very compassionate, and prescribed light physical therapy and massage. The facility he referred her to was associated with his practice.

A few weeks of therapy passed and the pain worsened. Kim was reporting more pain and discomfort now, then she had experienced just after the injury. Christian doctor didn't know what to think. She continued with the daily therapy sessions to no avail. Her condition was obviously worsening.

Aqua therapy was added to her care. Acupuncture was tried to no avail. A Tens unit was ordered. This little machine featured electrode pads that you attached to the painful area. Small electrical shocks or vibrations help disrupt the pain signals, break up scar tissue and provide relief. None of this was helping poor Kim. The surgeon considered surgery, as surgeons are prone to do. The therapist wanted more therapy, as therapists are prone to do. A chiropractor was called in. No improvement was noted. Eventually she was sent for an Electromyography. An EMG is a test where several electrodes are inserted into the muscle tissue and a neurologist observes the muscle activity while inserting the electrodes. It's painful. The electrodes are loaded with an electrical current that zaps the muscle. The test results came back hinting at neuropathy, or nerve pain often caused by Diabetes. Did Kim have diabetes? More tests were ordered. The results said no, she did not.

Off to see a neurologist, whom we'll call Dr. Handsome. Kim had a little crush on the good looking professional. He studied the previous results and dismissed them as fraudulent. No he didn't see signs of neuropathy, but was ordering a second EMG, to be certain. More pain was in store for Kim. She feared having this procedure done again and resisted. She was given Valium to take in preparation. It was still very painful and brought Kim to tears. It was deemed necessary, but it seemed so invasive. Causing pain to a person already suffering seemed an odd decision. Upon receiving the results of the second EMG, Dr. Handsome declared that she had no neuropathy and as a neurologist there was nothing else he could really do for her.

Finally on March 17, 2009, the theory that this may be Reflex Sympathetic Dystrophy was first floated. Christian doctor advised Kim to go home and study up on RSD via the internet. He warned her that she would not like what she found. I was away on business at the time, so Kim spent her weekend reading, crying and worrying about her future, alone. The internet was full of horror stories. This was lousy advice to give her right then. She would start her long journey with visions of horrible pain and no cure prominent in her mind.

When I returned home I was confronted with a dire prognosis and a very depressed wife. Kim had learned that the only effective treatments for RSD were those employed after early diagnosis, within two to three months. Obviously we had missed that window of opportunity. Five months had passed since her injury. She was well into the second stage of the disease and rapidly progressing to the third and final stage.

There appeared to be no real cure for those who were not diagnosed early.

RSD/CRPS

REFLEX SYMPATHETIC DYSTROPHY, ALSO KNOWN as Chronic Regional Pain Syndrome, is a rare, chronic (long-term) and progressive condition characterized by severe pain, inflammation and skin changes.

Patients often describe the pain as a burning sensation which affects arms, legs, hands or feet. It is most common in women between the ages of forty and sixty.

It is usually the result of some minor injury, like a broken bone or contusion. The severity of the pain is out of proportion to the original injury, for reasons not quite understood. As I understand it, the original pathway that sends pain signals to the brain is stuck open. Even though the injury has healed, the pain signals are still being sent. There are also very real symptoms that occur. Kim suffered with all of them.

Changes in skin temperature: the skin may be sweaty in some cases, or cold and clammy in other.

Changes in skin color: there may be blotches or streaks on the skin. Pink or blue tinges may appear.

Skin texture: the skin may turn thin and shiny.

Nails and hair: hair and nails may grow at unusual speed.

Joints: affected joints become stiff, painful and inflamed.

Mobility: the patient may have a harder and harder time using the affected limb.

Allodynia: the skin of the affected area becomes hyper-sensitive to touch. Even the lightest of clothing causes pain.

Over time, the affected limb can become cold and pale and undergo skin and nail changes as well as muscle spasms and tightening. Once these changes occur, the condition is often irreversible.

Historically, RSD was noticed during the Civil War in patients who had suffered a gunshot wound with damage to the median nerve. In 1867 the condition was known as causalgia from the Greek term meaning burning pain. The exact causes of RSD are still unclear. Patients in the later stage of RSD present with a pale, cold, painful and atrophic extremity. Patients at this point will also have osteoporosis. Kim would progress through all of the stages.

Before the accident, Kim was a very active professional. Her job required her to walk miles each day, often hustling to make a meeting or cater to the needs of some big shot. She would often work seventy hours or more per week. During race week, which was twice per year, she would log over one hundred hours, sleeping in the Green Room for a few hours each night. It was hectic, but she was very proud of her position. She had the long sculpted legs of an athlete. She relied on caffeine to keep her going, never letting the stress slow her down.

After the accident, she became trapped in a body that wouldn't cooperate. Her left leg quickly began to wither away. Pain was her constant companion. She was always a beautiful woman. I loved to be seen with her in public. There is nothing like having a tall, slender, head-turning blonde on your arm at a special event. But we started noticing changes. She wouldn't wear any clothing on her legs due to the extreme sensitivity. The blotches and streaks of color were clear to see. Her "little leg" as she called it, became noticeably thinner than her good leg. Her toenails grew malformed.

The little leg stiffened and she lost coordination. Balance became a problem. She told me it felt like a vise tightening a little each day on her leg. She would cry due to the bone crushing agony she was experiencing.

Meanwhile she had to get herself to therapy every day. I missed a lot of time at work taking her to various doctor's appointments. We didn't fully understand everything that was happening to her, but we knew that none of the treatments were helping. She became despondent and I felt helpless. I had no idea what to do.

We were newlyweds at the time. Our new life together held so much promise. We both had great jobs. We were both very healthy and relatively young. We were deeply in love and the future had seemed limitless for us. Now it was all being stolen away by a disease that we couldn't comprehend.

Nothing that was being said or done provided us with any hope.

THE EARLY DOCTORS

CHRISTIAN DOCTOR WAS CONVINCED NOW that Kim indeed had RSD. He told us her only option was to see a pain management specialist. She was stuck with this condition and it would probably get worse. Let's try to control the pain. He recommended us to Dr. Quack across town.

On her first visit with Dr. Quack, he quickly pronounced that she did not have RSD. He wasn't convinced that RSD even existed. His examination was brief and pointless. She left with a prescription for a mild narcotic painkiller.

It did nothing at all to relieve her pain. We called to make a second appointment in hopes of having her medication changed or adjusted. As she sat in the exam room waiting to see Dr. Quack, a nurse came in and escorted her out the back door. The doctor would not be seeing her today. Out front she noticed the locked doors and other patients milling about wondering what was going on. We never did find out what happened to him. This didn't speak well for the recommendation of Christian doctor.

Our second attempt with a pain management professional was with Dr. Senile. This older gentlemen appeared to have lost some of his higher cognitive functions. He did give her a stronger medication, but nothing much else. One day I had an idea. Back in my younger days as a baseball pitcher I had experience shoulder pain. Someone gave me something called DMSO (Dimethyl Sulfoxide). DMSO was a liquid originally used as a solvent to clean parts in factories. It was discovered that once arthritic workers were experiencing less pain and greater mobility after working with it. You rubbed it on the problem area, and over time your pain lessened and your mobility improved. It worked pretty well for me.

I mentioned it to Kim. We were willing to try most anything at this point. She called Dr. Senile and he said, "Sure, come on in and I'll give you a bottle." I drove the hour to pick it up and remembered a curious side effect. The liquid, once applied, gave you bad garlic breath. I warned Kim about this, but neither of us thought too much about it.

When I got home from work the next day, I entered into Garlic Hell. The whole house smelled very strongly of garlic. This wasn't just a simple case of garlic breath. Kim's entire body reeked of it. She almost had a fog around her as the pungent odor seeped from her pores. That was the last dose of DMSO for her. It took several days for our air quality to return to normal.

When we called to make the next appointment with Dr. Senile, we learned that he had suffered a stroke. No one knew when, or if he would return to his practice.

We were back to square one. Kim had no doctor, no relief, and no hope.

It was at this point that we were introduced to a "patient advocate". Up until now the worker's compensation insurance carrier had been patient. We'll call them the Big Z. They assigned a nurse to monitor Kim's care and to make recommendations. We felt we had no choice but to listen to her.

She set us up with yet another pain management specialist, our third. His office was two hours away, which became a major inconvenience for us. I'll call him Dr. Drill Sergeant. He was clearly an advocate of the No Pain No Gain school of thought. The patient advocate kept drilling him about RSD. "Does she really have it?" His examination was thorough and he wouldn't be rushed. He also had the records from all the previous doctors. Eventually he agreed with the diagnosis. You could visibly see the alleged advocate deflate.

He prescribed yet another new narcotic called Embeda. This one actually offered a bit of relief. He wanted Kim to perform regular exercise, see a chiropractor, and attend a different therapist. The advocate sent her to what turned out to be a "Work Hardening" program. Kim lasted one day and came home in excruciating pain.

We called our lawyer about this woman's intrusion into Kim's treatment. We were informed that we did not have to allow her into the doctor's office nor follow her recommendations on which provider to see.

Not knowing where else to turn, we continued to see Dr. Drill Sergeant. He was tough. Kim's not working hard enough. It's going to hurt anyway so just do it. He lacked any compassion whatsoever.

After no improvements were noted, he decided to give Kim some pain blocking injections. This was to be done under sedation, in the hospital. We drove the two hours on the appointed day and took our places in the waiting room. Kim hobbled to the water cooler and took a small sip of water. She was immediately called to the nurse's station. "I'm sorry ma'am, but we have to cancel your injections. You can't drink water before the procedure." There we were, two hours from home. There would be no relief today.

The drive home was a somber one. I was livid with the hospital, but tried hard to keep my emotions in check. Kim just sat with her head hung down. There was nothing to do but keep on keeping on.

Eventually we returned for the shots. Kim emerged numb from the waist down and a bit high. The drive home featured her telling me it was our day to bring snacks for the soccer match. There was no soccer match. In fact, neither of the kids was playing soccer at the time.

She seemed to be pain free on that drive. It was to be short-lived. As soon as the numbness wore off, the pain returned. The shots didn't work. We returned two more times, for two more rounds of shots. The outcome was the same. Dr. Drill Sergeant had no other tricks. He upped the Embeda and sent us to a chiropractor. He also prescribed another medication called Neurontin. This was supposed to help calm nerve pain. Over the course of several months he gradually increased her dose to thirty-six hundred milligrams per day. We later learned this was a ridiculously high amount.

Dr. Yacht was a nice enough fellow. He liked to brag about his big boat that he kept on the Jersey shore. He also drove a fancy BMW. His modus operandi was typical chiropractor fare. Kim went for treatments three times a week for months with no discernible improvement. Dr. Yacht decided to up his game. He started stringing up Kim in his traction machine. Picture a mid-evil torture device designed to stretch the spine millimeters at a time. Not surprisingly, this had a very negative effect on Kim's well being. The pain worsened. The other symptoms worsened. She was going downhill fast.

At this point we took it upon ourselves to try to get into John's Hopkins hospital in Baltimore, Maryland. We made enough phone calls until someone agreed to consult with Kim and suggest a course of treatment. After a lengthy exam and thorough study of her records, they offered one possible option. They wanted to insert a spinal cord stimulator. An electrode would be inserted into the spine. It would give off tiny vibrations to disrupt the pain signals being sent. First a trial would be done with an external controller. If the trial was a success, surgery would be performed to install the controller under her skin.

They sent us home with a DVD on the procedure, which included testimonials from happy patients. We did our own research. It appeared that the SCS was an option of last resort. Patients were not eligible unless all other options had failed. It had an alarming rate of complications, which usually meant additional surgery to adjust the electrode.

Our other physicians were not enthused about the idea. We felt we didn't have any other choice. After thinking it over we asked to be approved for the surgery and insertion of the Spinal Cord Stimulator. Our request was denied by the insurance company. Kim was willing to take the risk in hopes of any chance at all that it would help. Big Z was unwilling to pay for it. The option of last resort would not be available to us.

BECOMING A CAREGIVER

Back home things started falling apart. Kim couldn't perform the simplest tasks most of the time. She started to rely on me to help her to the bathroom and to help her bathe. Before all of this, I routinely worked sixty hours per week. Now I was showing up less than forty. My time was consumed with doctors' appointments, assisting Kim and housework.

I started noticing additional changes in Kim's behavior. She would grow sullen at times, more than just a bad mood. I couldn't blame her so I wrote it off to depression. Then things started to get bizarre. She began to sleepwalk on a regular basis. She forgot almost everything. I'd come home from work and listen to her stories. A few hours later I'd listen to the same stories again. If I told her that I'd already heard that, she'd get frustrated with herself. Sometimes I just didn't let on that I was hearing the same thing over again.

She couldn't sleep at night due to the pain. When she did go to bed, she would talk in her sleep and toss about violently for hours. I started sleeping in the spare bedroom. I wanted to be close to her, but I still had to work. My own lack of sleep was wearing me down.

One night I awoke to strange noises coming from my office area. I found Kim sitting at the computer, pretending to drive a car, while making driving noises. She was soaking wet. After guiding her back to bed I cleaned up the large water spill on my keyboard and papers.

I was worried that she could hurt herself while I was asleep. I trained myself to sleep very lightly so that I would wake at the slightest noise. This didn't leave me feeling particularly rested, but it was nothing compared to the pain Kim was experiencing. The medicines that her doctors were prescribing were fogging her brain, while doing little to lessen her pain. Occasionally she would say or do something that was hurtful to me. I could not respond. She was the one in pain.

I started doing some further research as a way to cure my feelings of helplessness. I fix things. I couldn't fix this and it was tearing me up. I was watching my wife fall into despair. I was watching her lose herself as the disease took control of her. We were no longer intimate in a physical way. I didn't want to cause her pain and her sleep patterns were extremely erratic. Things were spiraling out of control.

My first case study was the neurontin, also known as gabapentin. The list of side effects was alarming.

- Changes in behavior

- Memory problems

- Trouble concentrating

- Acting restless, hostile or aggressive

I was pretty sure that this drug was behind the changes in Kim's behavior. I waited for just the right time, when Kim was relatively coherent, to discuss the matter. We managed to make it through the conversation without much argument. She got a little light in her eyes at the knowledge of the drug's causing some of these problems. Together we decided to wean her off of it. We never told Dr. Drill Sergeant. We filled her new prescriptions each month, and gradually decreased her dosage until she quit taking it all together.

Her pain did not improve but her disposition got much better. Her mind cleared somewhat and she started to fight back. I found an Internet message board where she could talk with fellow RSD sufferers. This was good therapy for a while. She was not alone. She ended up encouraging others to keep fighting. This was our first tiny ray of hope.

Next I started researching alternative treatments for RSD. There were hyperbaric chamber treatments, homeopathic cures, ketamine comas, and any number of bizarre claims to a cure. I started rising an hour earlier each day in order to read medical journals and clinical trials. I investigated cost and availability of each of the proposed cures.

I would mention each to Kim in our nightly discussions. We didn't have a plan yet but we were desperately seeking one. The sessions with Dr. Yacht were eventually discontinued. We only saw Dr. Drill Sergeant to get new prescriptions each month. We had to look in some other direction, but what was it?

The most promising treatment was called a ketamine coma. The patient was flooded with ketamine, a highly hallucinogenic drug used to tranquilize large animals. Kids use it to get high, when they can steal it from veterinary offices. Along with the ketamine, an anti-hallucinogen is administered. The patient is kept in a coma for a week or more, literally to prevent them from going insane. It has actually shown great promise. Unfortunately it is not available in the United States. We would have to travel to Germany or Mexico. It was also very expensive and not covered by any American insurance.

The second most promising treatment also involved ketamine. A clinic in Tampa, Florida offers outpatient infusions over a month's time. The dose is much lower than the coma option, but given over a longer period of time. They do not accept insurance and you are expected to pay in cash, up front. This option did not have as good a success rate as the coma option, but seemed much less risky. It was also conceivably affordable for us.

I put the ketamine infusion clinic on my mental list of options and set out to find us a new doctor. The Internet can be a wonderful thing. I eventually Googled up a pain management specialist, not too far from home, with many glowing reviews from happy patients.

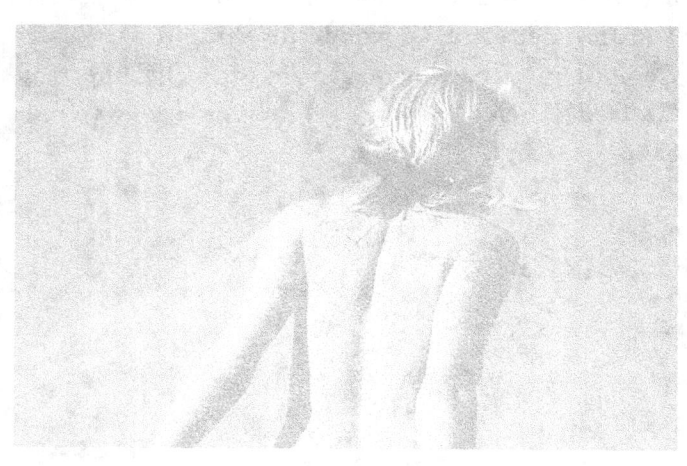

THE WITCH DOCTOR

WE ARRIVED AT OUR FIRST appointment with this our fourth pain management specialist, to be greeted by a tiny little Indian man. Without provocation he assured us that he was a Hindu, and not a Muslim. He skin was dark as coal along with his hair and his eyes. Something was wrong with one hand which he hid underneath a glove. He had remarkably white teeth that shined out at you as he constantly smiled. He seemed a very happy fellow. He spoke much like Apu of "The Simpsons", only harder to understand. "Would you like a Slurpee straw with that?"

His nurse was not really a nurse, rather just an assistant. She claimed to be a Wiccan, of the white magic variety. His operating theater was in a house. It was just the two of them doling out happy pills to desperate patients. We certainly qualified as desperate, so we were in for the ride.

His very first order of business was to prescribe Marinol, a synthetic marijuana in pill form. He sent me out to fill the prescription while he took Kim into his office. I returned to hear about the benefits of eating a teaspoon of tumeric each day. He then went on to explain the healing properties of cactus to us. You eat it he said. By this time the one painkiller that seemed to help, Embeda, had been discontinued. He prescribed straight codeine, which turned out to be nearly impossible to fill.

He scheduled Kim for an epidural injection in the following weeks. Not the same lame pain blocking shots that didn't work, but an injection directly into the spinal cord, like they use during childbirth.

We left feeling uplifted. He was so enthusiastic that it was contagious. We bought tumeric and cactus on the way home. That night we shared our cautious optimism. He might be a Witch Doctor, but he was our Witch Doctor.

By the time we returned for the epidural, some of Kim's enthusiasm had worn off. She couldn't stand to swallow the tumeric, and eating cactus just didn't agree with her. She was visibly nervous about taking a needle in her spine, in the back room of a house, with a white Wiccan holding her hand. She told the Witch Doctor she hated needles and that she was afraid. He said he would numb the area with a cooling spray and she wouldn't feel a thing. The spray ran down her crack and onto a most delicate area. Kim squealed that she had a frozen hooha. The Witch Doctor began to sing to her. "Well, here's to you, Mrs. Robinson..." My God what had we gotten ourselves into?

A few minutes later, the Wiccan faux nurse came out to get me. She took me to the Witch Doctor who asked me to please sit with my wife and monitor her for a while. I asked what should I be looking for? He said she may hallucinate, and if she does he can't let her leave until she comes out of it. He had injected her spinal cord with ketamine!

I approached Kim with trepidation. I asked her if she felt okay. She said, "I feel F@#King great!" (This was totally out of character for her). She couldn't feel her legs, she couldn't walk, but she felt just fine, thank you very much. Finally she was cleared to leave. With the help of a walker and a Wiccan I was able to get her into our truck. She smiled and laughed all the way home. I wasn't sure what to think, but it was nice to see her smile. It was the first time I'd heard her laugh in over a year.

When we made it home, she was completely unable to walk. I positioned the truck with the passenger door close to our entrance. Then I put her in a fireman's carry and lugged her into the house. She needed to pee. I carried her to the bathroom and got her in position. Then I carried her back to the living room and plopped her in the recliner. I set her up with anything she wanted. She had the TV remote, a big glass of water, and her favorite comforter. She was at peace for the first time in a long time. We both loved the Witch Doctor.

The effects of the ketamine lasted about one week. Kim was able to get up and move around on her own. She did some dishes and even a little laundry. Soon enough, though, the despicable pain returned in full force. She was now taking Marinol every day. Mixing it with a glass of wine, she would catch a nice buzz and forget her pain for a few hours. The Witch Doctor said, "So what if you get high? If it makes you feel good, so much the better." We spent every evening getting pleasantly numb together.

Then came the oral ketamine. The Witch Doctor gave Kim a needleless syringe filled with ketamine. He instructed her to shoot it into the roof of her mouth. He couldn't give the injections too close together, but this would tide her over. The result was a deep stupor which I could not enter. She called it going into the K-hole. While she was under the influence of ketamine, she had no pain. It did nothing long-term, though. Once it wore off she was back to writhing on the floor. Between the Marinol, the ketamine epidurals, and the oral ketamine, she was pretty highed up most of the time. I briefly considered toying with her by making up some little pink elephants and dancing them in front of her eyes. Thank God I never followed through with that plan. So she was high most of the time. It was better than the alternative, but we both knew this couldn't go on forever.

As much as we appreciated the Witch Doctor and the Wiccan, his unconventional approach wasn't much better than the early doctors' at fixing the problem.

(Witch Doctor was a former associate of Christian Doctor. They had a falling out. If Christian Doctor would have sent us directly to the Witch Doctor during the early stages, we believe the disease's progression could have been halted.)

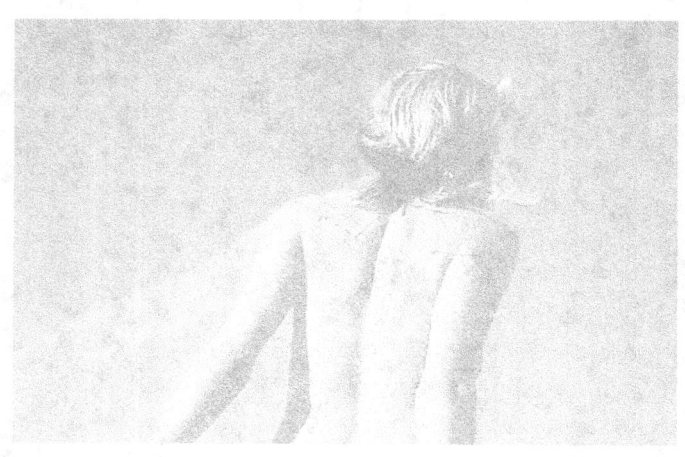

LAWYERS, DRUGS, AND MONEY

OUR LIVES WERE REVOLVING AROUND Kim's drugs. Soon they would revolve around lawyers, and the prospect of money. We hadn't given any thought to getting money out of this deal. We only wanted Kim to be healed. For her to have a normal life and for us to return to the promise we once had as a newly married couple was all we could hope for.

Big Z, however, was tiring of paying for expensive medications. They didn't like much paying the workman's compensation either. It was becoming clear that this was going to be a long-term, if not permanent, situation. They were desperate to get out. Their lawyer, we'll call him The Dick, filed to terminate benefits. Our lawyer, we'll call her Bulldog, immediately shot back a request for permanent disability payment. She was a petite, frail little lady who had shown no signs of a killer instinct in our previous dealings. We had even tried to replace her early in the process. As it turned out, that would have been a big mistake.

We scheduled a hearing with the Workers' Compensation Board. We had no idea what to expect. We could lose benefits, get a settlement and continued benefits, or anyplace in between. When the day arrived I thought Kim would break down. She was using a cane to get around at this point. Wearing pants was out of the question due to the increased skin sensitivity. She wore a very light skirt on a cold day. She had lost a lot of weight and she looked pathetic entering the boardroom. She fidgeted in her chair and was clearly nervous and uncomfortable throughout the proceedings. She decided not to take her Marinol before the hearing, in order to keep a clear head. I could see she was in intense pain. The added stress was taking its toll.

The Dick didn't have much to offer as justification for stopping her medical treatments. He offered up a career specialist who testified that she could find a job for Kim. The listings were pathetic, exemplified by a four hour-per-day job in a prison facility ninety minutes from our home. Bulldog blew this lady away on the witness stand. When the witness offered a position with Wells Fargo, as a loan consultant, Bulldog read off a list of drugs that Kim was taking daily. "Do you want your affairs handled by someone taking codeine, ketamine, and synthetic marijuana?"

The prospect of Kim's returning to work was dismissed by the board unanimously. We moved on to compensation. The Dick had made Kim see their "independent" doctor for evaluation. Bulldog had her see our own "independent" physician. Our guy was a genius who made their guy look like a fool. We took a break on Kim's behalf. She shuffled out of the boardroom and sat outside in the hall. I held her hand. I hugged her. I felt as if my support was so little, but it was all I had. We were just being led around by lawyers at this point, out of control of our own destiny. The Witch Doctor gave a deposition, which was read to the court. It only succeeded in confusing matters. No one really understood what he was saying. Bulldog snapped and growled at every turn. She shredded The Dick to pieces in our opinion.

Finally the hearing was over, with no determination given. We would have to wait for a verdict. It was a very long ride home. Kim was at a low point. She didn't care how it turned out. Whatever would happen, would happen. I took her home, fed her the meds, and filled her glass with wine.

Meanwhile the codeine was getting harder and harder to find. There are so many newer narcotics on the market today that few pharmacies stock it anymore. We had a list of twenty drug stores within a one-hour drive, with phone numbers and addresses. Each time we got a new prescription we'd start calling the list.

Kim started to develop an immunity to it. It just wasn't helping much with the pain. The Witch Doctor advised her to double up on the number of pills she was taking. This caused her to run out too soon. When she tried to fill another prescription, the pharmacy threw her out. They accused her of being a drug seeker, and threatened to call the police. Kim called me in tears. She was humiliated. She was also out of pain meds.

We called the Witch Doctor and he rewrote the prescription. After calling half the list we finally were able to fill it. Again, our lives revolved around Kim's drugs.

The stress of the Workers' Compensation Board hearing, the lawyers, the paperwork, and the uncertainty as to the outcome was too much for Kim to handle. She started to develop severe nausea, vomiting a dozen times per day. She lost more weight. She became very weak and frail. The vomiting could come at any time or any place. She kept plastic bags in the glove box so she could vomit while riding to the doctor's appointments. She stopped eating.

We went back to the Witch Doctor with a new problem. He prescribed an anti-nausea medication, adding to the long list of pills she was already taking. The Marinol was also supposed to help with her appetite. It was often given to cancer patients undergoing chemo to combat nausea and increase appetite. Neither seemed to help with Kim's nausea. The vomiting continued at an alarming pace. She was loosing enamel on her teeth. She'd brush them a dozen times per day. She lost all interest in food.

There was no therapy being given at this time. Kim was simply taking tons of pills, lying around the house and wasting away. Her little leg was shockingly small. It was really hard to see the daylight at the end of the tunnel. What good would a cash settlement do at this point?

I started considering that very question. I spoke with Bulldog about it. She seemed confident that we'd continue having our medical expenses paid and would most likely get some amount of additional compensation for Kim's injury. Maybe we could use it for one of those ketamine treatments. The clinic in Tampa seemed the most likely option. I went back to the Internet to further research the topic. The Tampa clinic offered roughly a fifty percent chance of immediate relief, with a long-term success rate of twenty to thirty percent. Some patients were seemingly cured, but later had the RSD reoccur. Some stayed cured forever, while others saw no long-term benefit from the treatments.

Somehow this led me to start thinking about moving to Florida.

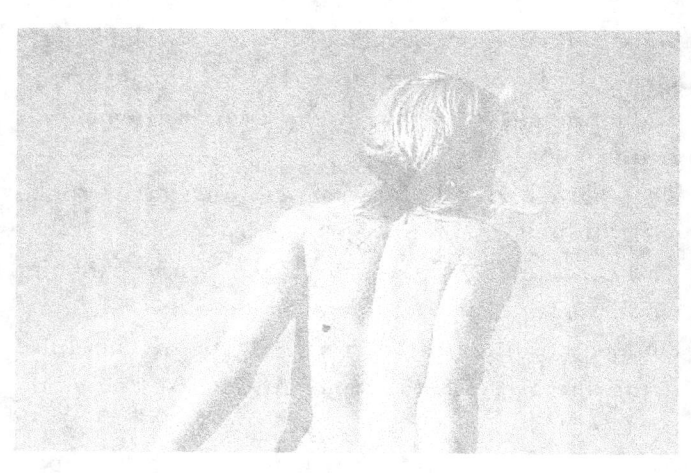

A DREAM AMID
THE CHAOS

B Y SHEER COINCIDENCE, MY COMPANY had
a job opening in Winter Haven, Florida.
Winter Haven is a short drive from Tampa. I
applied and was asked to fly down for an interview.
I was going to have to leave Kim by herself for a
few days and was worried about that. Also, her
grandfather was in very poor health and not expected
to last much longer. The situation couldn't get any
more stressful. Kim went to stay with a good friend
and had an aunt close by to help if necessary.

The interview in Florida went extremely well. I
had visions of collecting a bit of cash from the Big
Z, moving to Florida, getting Kim treatment, and
starting life anew. Before I could get home, Kim's
grandfather died. She was basically raised by him,
and loved and admired him greatly. He was a special
man to all, but no one was closer to him than his
little Kimmie. I returned in time for the funeral, and
guided a very depressed wife through the ceremonies.

Each time we thought things couldn't get any worse, we were proven wrong.

The job opportunity in Winter Haven didn't work out. I was stunned because I knew I nailed the interview. No word from Bulldog yet. I started to hate leaving the house each day to go to work. It turned out that my company had purchased another business in Florida, and some restructuring was in order to combine the two units. Would I be willing to go to West Palm Beach for a job? This was to be a working interview. I'd spend a week in Florida, working with the staff of the newly purchased company. I was instructed to take my wife along, all expenses paid.

This couldn't have come at a better time. We had snow on the ground at home. Kim had developed a real aversion to the cold, and I really needed a change. A little vacation for Kim in Florida sounded like just the ticket. While I worked during the day she took frequent advantage of the hot tub. She would lie poolside and read, soaking in the warm Florida sun. In the evenings we'd go out to a nice restaurant, have a few drinks and relax together. Her color improved, her mood improved and she even reported a slight decrease in her pain level. Five days in the Florida sun, far from the snow or the courtroom, had been therapeutic. This moving to Florida idea might not have been so crazy after all.

Back at home we started talking about it every night. We'd had enough of the cold and snow. We both believed that our stay in Florida had benefitted Kim. Having a goal and dreaming of a new life in the sunshine lifted both our spirits. I started working on downsizing our stuff to prepare for the move. I sold one of our two boats and got rid of a bunch of stuff in the garage. We were really excited about the possibilities.

Then I found out that I did not get the job. It was like a hard punch to the gut. All of our enthusiasm rushed out of us like the air from a popped balloon. I've never been so down in all of my life. I couldn't begin to imagine how Kim felt. I spent the next several days shoveling out from a massive blizzard that hit the Mid-Atlantic. I hated shoveling snow. I hated my job. I hated doctors and lawyers and this damn disease. I had failed to save us. I had let Kim down and I hated that the most. I started complaining to her every night about my stupid job, the stupid customers, and the stupid employees. Now she was my therapist as much as I was hers. It was not a happy time in the life of Kim and Ed.

We added tequila to our nightly drinking routine. I'd go to bed hammered and not hear Kim get up in the night. She got into all sorts of mischief while I lay stoned in bed. I'd drag my sorry ass to work in the morning to face another day at a job I hated. We filled prescriptions for more and more drugs. Kim's health was back to its lowest point again. There seemed to be no way out. Our lives together were swirling down the drain. We were helpless to stop it.

I didn't understand how Kim kept from considering suicide throughout all of this. She was down, but she never threw in the towel. She simply continued to persevere. We never lost our love for one another either. We spent so much time together. Every moment seemed precious. We discussed our inner fears, shared our memories and consistently professed our love to each other. I believe we were closer than most couples, maybe because of our circumstance. We had a song that we listened to together:

"She said, it'll work out. I have no regrets. You've shown me a life that I'll never forget.

She said, I'll be there, till the light, dies in your eyes."

It made me start to cry every time I heard it. I couldn't love her more, but I felt that I wasn't doing enough. What could I do? My thoughts returned to Florida. I wanted to take Kim to a warm tropical beach and let her lie in the sun. I wanted her to forget about doctors and lawyers. There had to be a way.

I spent a few days reflecting on our situation. If we didn't do something, Kim was going to die. I couldn't let that happen. I kept telling myself, "You're a smart guy, you fix things. Come up with something." I took stock of our finances. We had some cash in the bank from the sale of the boat. We also spent very little and the checking account was fairly fat. We no longer went out to eat or to concerts or the movies. We just stayed home, locked up in the house drinking tequila and popping pills. All Kim's medical expenses were being paid by Big Z.

The plan slowly took shape. Let's pay off our debt, save a bunch of money, get rid of our stuff, and take off for Florida. I brought this idea to Kim. Quit your job? What will we do for money? I told her we'd live off savings for a while. It would work out. I didn't think she had a high level of confidence in this plan, but she trusted in me. Somehow, it would indeed work out.

Now I had something I could do to combat the plight we were in. I could take action. I felt that I'd found my purpose. I was not going to be an innocent bystander to my wife's death. If she did die, I was going to provide her with some happiness on the way out. I think Kim sensed all of this. She didn't bring it up, instead allowing me to do my thing. She probably thought the whole thing was a silly dream at the time. I was determined to show her that it was not.

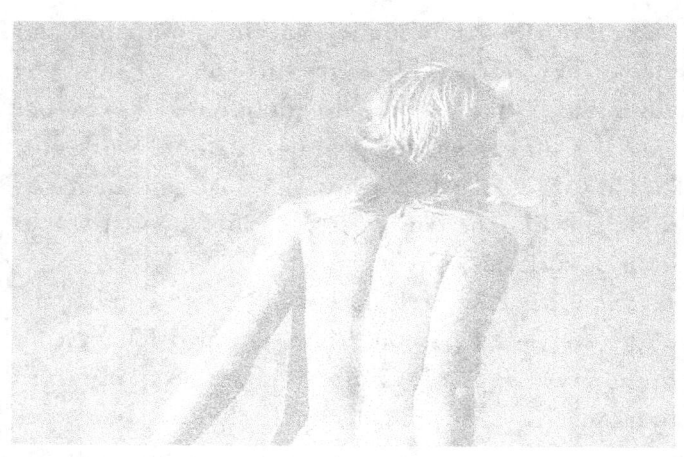

TAKING ACTION

I CONTINUED TO CARE FOR KIM's needs as best I could. I tried to make sure she had everything she needed. I tried to make her comfortable. I did the laundry, washed the dishes, cleaned the house, and focused on our finances. Kim began doing some light stretching exercises on her own. We feared she would lose all use of her little leg eventually. She quit taking the oral ketamine, but continued with the epidurals. These would give her some measure of relief for shorter and shorter periods of time.

I had to raise money quickly. I started having my employer deposit directly into our savings account. I had them deduct as much as I thought we could afford. When I saw that we could manage okay on the reduced income, I upped the deposit even more. I eliminated all frivolous spending. I'm not here to tell you how to manage your own money, but suffice it to say we all spend way too much on things we don't really need. This was an important lesson I learned through this process. It would serve us well in the future.

I took the money from the sale of the boat and paid off my truck. This freed up four hundred dollars each month, which all went into savings. I paid off one credit card after another. Each time I'd see extra money in checking as a result, I'd transfer it to savings. At each milestone on the bank ledger, I'd gleefully tell Kim how much we had saved. I became obsessed with saving money and growing the account balance. I started selling off possessions. Out went the tools. Away went the fishing rods.

This led to a whole new obsession, getting rid of stuff. I started giving things away. Any needy acquaintance was freely given something they needed, like a sofa or Christmas decorations. We actually gave the sofa to the white Wiccan. Between selling and giving I completely emptied our previously over-full garage. Kim just eyed me during this time, watching me come and go with bags for Goodwill. She didn't have any interest in giving away all of her stuff. She concentrated on adjusting her meds and keeping up with the stretching. The stretching didn't seem to help, but we convinced ourselves that it was preventing her from getting worse.

During this time we grew fond of island music. We had this dream of living on a tropical island, so it was nice to supplement it with songs about the island life. It really did help to keep our spirits up. It may have been while listening to a song about boats, that a brand new thought entered my brain. What about living on a boat? Before we were married, Kim and I had chartered a yacht in the British Virgin Islands. I proposed to her there, on our first night aboard. We spent a week cruising the crystal clear Caribbean Sea, hopping from one tropical island to the next. It was the greatest week of our lives.

"Hey Kim," I said one day. "How about I quit my job and we'll go live on a boat? She looked me dead in the eye and said, "I'm game." I couldn't believe it. I thought she would say I was crazy. God bless her. There would be lots of details to work out. Her condition didn't really seem to blend well with a nautical lifestyle. On the other hand, we could live cheaply in warm, sunny places. Both of us were raised around boats and loved the ocean. We were alike in a lot of ways, but our love of the sea was our biggest common denominator. I loved her more in that moment than I'd ever thought possible. I had to pull this off, for her.

To my growing list of duties I added research about living aboard. I researched boats. I researched places to live on boats. I learned all the technical aspects of boat operation and maintenance. I already had a captain's license and a deep familiarity with many of the aspects of a life at sea. I was only sleeping four hours a night. I read so many books and magazines and Internet articles that I had anchors and windlasses in my dreams. I started showing boats to Kim on the Internet. We would spend hours looking at boats and deciding what we liked and didn't like. It was a nice distraction for us both.

I was still going to that job every day, but it didn't seem so bad now. I had to save money. The job was a means to an end. Kim's pain was never far from my mind, but I was feeling like I was doing something to help. I kept working and I kept saving. I kept caring for Kim and she kept on staying alive. She never gave up. She really had no reason to think things would ever get better for her, but she refused to give in. She was my hero. I have serious doubts that I could have handled myself as well as she did in the same situation. Her strength amazes me to this day.

Finally we got the call from Bulldog. Our lawyer was pleased to announce that we had won the case against Big Z. Kim's medical expenses would continue to be covered, and we would be awarded a modest settlement for her injuries. Let me take a minute to explain our experience with workman's comp in the state of Delaware. You don't get rich from it, no matter how severe your injury. Delaware's laws are designed to protect the employer as much as the employee. They have a monetary value placed on each body part. Say you lose an entire leg. It has a value. We'll call it one hundred thousand dollars. If you lost half your leg, you'd get fifty thousand, and so on. The board determined that Kim had lost fifty percent use of her leg, so we'd be getting a check. Bulldog would keep one third. It wasn't much considering how much suffering Kim had endured, but they don't pay for pain and suffering.

We were relieved that this particular episode in our ordeal was over. Anything that reduced the stress on Kim was a good thing. She felt vindicated in her battle with Big Z. She was happy that Bulldog had taken down The Dick. We'd have to wait for months to get paid, and it did nothing to relieve her pain, but it was a victory nonetheless. Three cheers for Kim!

Now I needed to take a real hard, honest look at our money situation. We had a nice amount in savings, but not enough to live on for very long. I also had a nice amount in my 401K, which I had been contributing the maximum amount to. Add these two amounts to the settlement check, and the dream was almost feasible. I thought long and hard. I agonized over it. Throwing away my career and risking it all didn't seem very wise to me. Then I thought of Kim. I started this obsession with money in order to save her. There was no turning back now.

I was going to pull out all the money, get rid of the rest of our stuff, and take Kim to paradise to live on a boat. It was a crazy thing to do, I'll admit. Once the decision was made though, I had a huge load off my shoulders. When I broke the news to her she was overjoyed. We hugged and laughed and smiled and enjoyed a brief moment of happiness in each other's arms.

It wouldn't be long before the outside world crept back in to our dreams.

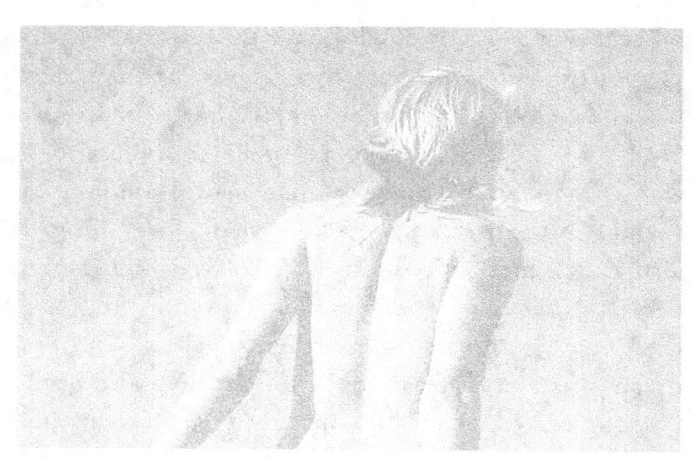

SPIES AT HOME
AND ON THE ROAD

W E LIVED IN A SMALL, private community well off the main road. You left the state road, took the county road, then drove down a dirt road to get to our home. It was a well-wooded area with no street lights. The seclusion was welcomed during Kim's ordeal. We didn't want to be around other people much. We didn't talk to the neighbors much either. We just wanted to be left alone, safe inside our home. We had plenty of our own problems to deal with.

Somewhere along the way, Kim started to become paranoid about being watched. She told me that she could feel eyes upon her when I wasn't home. She felt like we were being followed when we went somewhere. We even joked about it. If we were out and a small plane would fly over, we'd say "There goes Big Z." We asked Bulldog about this possibility and she told us that there was a high probability that investigators would watch Kim, especially if she left the house. I understand the need for this in some situations. We've all seen the videos of some guy who claimed to have a bad back. The private detective will film him working under the table, carrying shingles up a ladder. There are too many instances of someone collecting disability while pursuing a new career in MMA fighting these days.

But Kim? I hate to say it but she was a cripple. Her infirmity had been proven before the Workers' Compensation Board. She could only get around without assistance on her best days, usually right after an injection. She wasn't going to be climbing any ladders or entering a fight ring anytime soon. The thought that Big Z may have hired spies to keep an eye on her seemed preposterous. It was not.

Later we got copies of the reports that the investigators sent to Big Z. They had placed a man somewhere on a neighboring property to spy on Kim many times. Often they would sit in the cold for eight hours and never catch a glimpse of her. Sometimes they would report that she came out and sat on the deck for ten minutes then went back inside. They never saw her carry a load of laundry or mow the grass or give any indication that she was a malingerer. They reported on my comings and goings. *A white male in his late forties was seen entering the driveway with a canoe in the back of a white pickup truck.* (It was a kayak.)

Kim's intuition was spot-on, though. She sensed that they were out there, and she was right. Have I told you she's an amazing woman yet? The problem now, though, was that we were prisoners in our own home. We never knew if we were being watched. The curtains stayed closed. How much did they see before we were alerted to their presence? With all of the many problems that Kim was forced to cope with, this was too much. She was being violated all over again by the evil forces of Big Z.

We later learned that they followed us when we left the house. They followed us to Walmart. They followed us to doctor's appointments. They tailed us to McDonalds. We began to keep an eye out for them. Every car behind us was suspicious. If we thought we were being tailed, we'd try to lose them. We'd pull into a gas station or take a road we hadn't intended to take in order to flush them out. In later reports the investigator admitted to calling off the chase occasionally because he thought we were on to him.

It was all quite maddening. It certainly did nothing to help Kim. Big Z's main interest was to stop paying her medical bills, not to get her healed. I've seen movies about the greed and ignorance of major insurance companies, but I never thought it could happen to us. I wonder how much money they wasted spying on an invalid? To what lengths would they go? As time passed we would find out. The lengths they went to would lead to a major turning point in our lives.

Now I was more determined than ever to take Kim far, far away. Our plan to escape would shield her from the prying eyes of hired snoops.

The added stress of constant surveillance was having a negative effect on Kim's well-being. This was not surprising, as stress seemed to be a major trigger for her pain. When we met she was just shy of six feet tall and carried one hundred and forty pounds quite well. She was trim, but she was also toned. There was not an ounce of fat on her. Now she weighed less than one twenty. Her bones started to protrude through her skin. Her once smooth skin was now blotched and streaked. Her hair started to fall out. What remained was very thin and dull.

She could manage to brush her teeth, or comb her hair, but she no longer took much care of her appearance. She was forced to dress in light, loose fitting clothes. She still vomited many times a day. She saw no point in makeup unless we had a doctor's appointment. It was painful to see her this way. When we would talk in the evenings though, I could still see the woman I loved inside her. Her eyes would still light up if I said something funny or clever. She was attentive to me in the ways that she could be. She listened to me. She understood me. We continued to share our dream. I'm pretty sure it was that dream that held us together.

She needed to hang on while I pulled it all together. It gave her something to look forward to. It kept me going as well. Living on a boat in paradise seemed awesome, but I wouldn't do it without the woman I loved.

As one final testament to the fact that we would follow through, I gave my boss notice that I was leaving, one full year in advance. I set a firm departure date. I told everyone whom I knew what our plans were. I couldn't back out now.

We spent that final year hoarding cash like misers. We steadily worked on divesting ourselves of all our possessions. Kim got with the program and discovered how freeing it was. We were going to do this. It didn't seem real but it was happening.

We had those who doubted us. There were some who pronounced us fools. Most didn't understand why we would do such a thing with Kim in her condition. Many of them never understood what was really going on with this disease they never heard of. She lost at least one close friend who talked behind her back, questioning just how hurt she really was. Kim struggled with this often. It was hard to explain her mysterious illness. Those people didn't see what she went through behind our walls. I saw. We also were given encouragement by some of our close friends. It was exciting, but it was all so uncertain. In spite of this horrible disease that had stricken Kim, even through all her pain, she was willing to take a leap of faith with me. We would face the unknown together. We'd figure out a way to ease her pain. We were moving onto a boat in paradise.

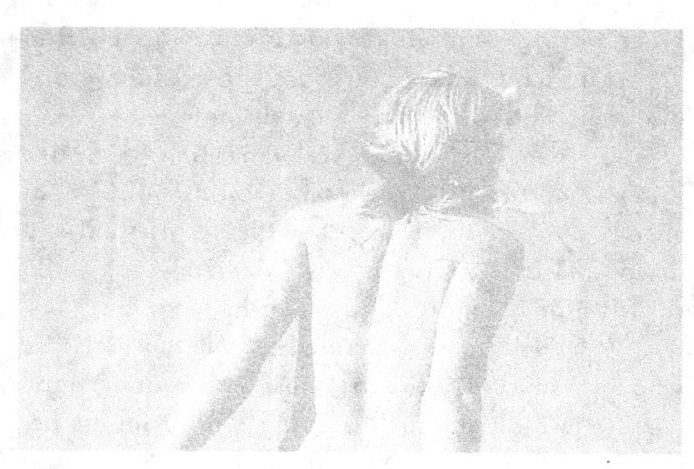

TAKING THE LEAP

WE SPENT THE LAST NIGHT in our home with nothing but a blow-up mattress. The truck was packed with what few meager belongings remained, mostly clothes. We had said our tearful goodbyes. Kim was well supplied with medications. All that was left to do was to drive away.

A few days after Christmas in 2010, we departed for the unknown. Any fears that remained were overwhelmed by the sheer feeling of freedom. We had no debt, no jobs, and no outside stress. We still had that giant monkey on Kim's back, but we had faith that it would all work out. You can't imagine how uplifting it was to have zero commitments. We were flooded with hope for the future for the first time in years. We had no thoughts of spies in the bushes as we drove down I-95 towards Florida.

We took our time, stopping often for Kim to stretch her legs. We stayed in hotels along the way. We spent a few days in the sun and sand at Cocoa Beach. On January 3, 2011, we arrived at our destination. There was a boat we thought we might buy in Punta Gorda. We rented a luxurious condo complete with hot tub. The boat shopping didn't work out as smoothly as we planned. We ended up staying in that condo for two months before finally moving aboard our new boat. We named her *Leap of Faith*.

We moved aboard her on the first of March. Two months in the sun and in the hot tub had slightly improved Kim's condition. No one else would notice, but I could tell. There was a tiny change in her disposition. She was still struggling mightily with pain. She still didn't eat much, and when she did a vomiting episode wouldn't be far behind. She was walking a little better, and a little more. I hoped that this trend would continue.

One night I took her out to a fancy restaurant on the water. Kim ordered the stone crabs, a Florida delicacy. Before her meal arrived she rushed to the ladies' room. She was so overcome with nausea that she couldn't eat a bite. We apologized to the waitress and took our meals to go. We obviously weren't out of the woods yet.

The next morning while she slept, I prepared her an omelet made with scrumptious Florida stone crab and expensive cheese. She ate like a ravenous lion. She declared this the best omelet ever, by far. I replied that it ought to be, it only cost thirty-five dollars. We got a good laugh out of that and she kept the omelet down. I hoped this trend wouldn't continue.

We couldn't afford thirty-five dollar-omelets every day. Bu if it was discovered that stone crab omelets cured RSD, I'd gladly buy them for every meal.

We eased into the live-aboard life slowly. Kim wanted to do so much more than she was capable of. She wanted to clean and to organize, like any woman with a new home would. As we settled in, we realized that the small confines were actually an asset to Kim. Everything on the boat was just a few steps away, and she could hold on to something anywhere she went. Maybe this wasn't such a dumb idea after all.

We started making new friends on the docks at the marina, and everyone was very helpful. We had a swimming pool, beaches nearby, and lots of sunshine. Kim began to socialize with the ladies while I worked on the boat. We enjoyed happy hour gatherings with our new friends. We sat and watched the sunset together every night.

Life was good in Kim and Ed's world, but we still hadn't made much progress in getting her healed. She was still in considerable pain. She went to great lengths to hide it from our neighbors and marina staff, but I knew. We had successfully made the leap from our old life to a sunny new one.

Now it was time to rejoin the fight. It was time to put Kim's treatment front and center. We were on our way, but we weren't there yet.

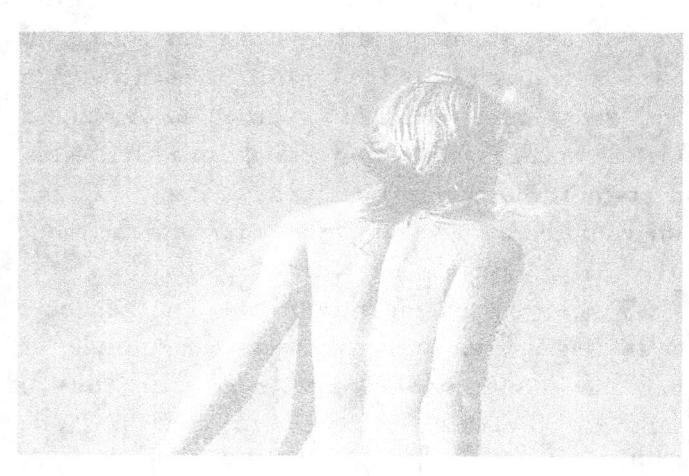

THE ROBOT DOCTOR

WE HAD MADE ARRANGEMENTS FOR a new doctor for Kim in Florida, before we ever left our old home. This would be our fifth pain management specialist. It would also be our last. We'll call him Robot Doctor. The day came to make our first appointment and Kim grew nervous. We were both pretty disgusted with doctors in general by this point. We could only hope that this one would be different.

When we arrived Kim was instructed to give a urine sample. They wanted to make sure she wasn't using non-prescription drugs. She wasn't. While waiting for the results Kim had to rush to the restroom, which was right next to the waiting room and nurses station. We could all hear what was going on in there. A wave of nausea had overcome her. There was a pattern to her discomfort. Stress was bad.

When she exited the restroom a nurse approached her with an insulting tone of voice. "Are you withdrawing?" She was sneering at Kim like she was some kind of low-life druggie. Kim explained that all the pills made her sick. I could see that she was taken aback by the nurse's manner. She didn't need this accusation during the first few minutes in a new doctor's office. This wasn't boding well for our experience with a new doctor.

In the exam room a different nurse treated Kim kindly. She took her blood pressure, which was way up. She took all her vital signs, patient history, etc. We gave her a list of all the current medications Kim was on. When she got to Marinol, she said "Oh no, we don't give that here." She stacked all the forms into a file and left the room. We just looked at each other. Things weren't starting off very well at all.

Finally the Robot Doctor arrived. He asked a few questions, did a minimal exam, and started to write prescriptions. There was no idle chatter, no bedside manner, no smiles, or even any appearance of concern. He did relent and allow the Marinol. We were scheduled for an injection in a few weeks. Robot Doctor informed us that there would be no ketamine, only steroid injections. We shrugged and left to find a pharmacy. "Well, that kind of sucked," I said. Kim more than agreed. She didn't like the doctor. She didn't like the nurses. It was not a promising experience.

With all of the excitement of our move and the new boat purchase, we'd forgotten just how frustrating modern medicine could be. It was a total reality check for us both. We still had a big problem, even though we had taken that leap. We couldn't run away from Kim's illness, or her pain. They would be with us wherever we went.

When we returned for Kim's first injection things went okay. Robot Doctor didn't speak much. There were no pleasantries. He did play nice music in the injection room, according to Kim. He was gentle and didn't cause her much pain. I never saw him. We drove back to the marina without saying a whole lot. I parked and had Kim wait in the truck while I went to the marina office. They sent a dockhand out in a golf cart and together we got her seated. He took her down the dock to our boat. Then we all shared an awkward moment as the two of us lowered her down on deck. He had his hands in some sensitive areas, not by choice but out of necessity. He couldn't help it. Kim felt embarrassed for him, not for herself. She'd been groped a hundred times by doctors over the past several years. No big deal if a dockhand touched her ass helping her on the boat.

We continued this routine for the next several months. Whenever she got a shot, we'd call for the golf cart and manhandle her onto the boat. I think the dock hands may have argued over who got to assist the lovely Miss Kim. The shots started to help a bit over time. Not dramatically so, but they gave her a week or two of relief. She was still sick to her stomach all the time, but the really severe fits of agonizing pain were less frequent. Any improvement, no matter how small, was welcomed.

Robot Doctor never got any friendlier. We complained about the nausea. He didn't care. We complained about her weight loss. He didn't care. Come in, get your prescriptions. Come back in two weeks and get your shot. Rinse and repeat. We couldn't tell if he even remembered who Kim was from appointment to appointment. One time Robot Doctor was not available for our appointment. Substitute Doctor listened to Kim's complaints. He changed the narcotic from a morphine derivative to something called Nucynta. This medicine was designed to treat severe pain. It still carried the same side effects, including nausea, dizziness, constipation, and sedation, but they were supposed to be less severe. The nurses did get friendlier. Once they realized that Kim wasn't a junkie, they treated her with more kindness. One of them overheard her weight loss discussion with the Robot and returned to offer Kim advice on making healthy smoothies that were easy to digest. We took her advice and started making smoothies. The nurses felt sorry for Kim and sometimes looked at her with pity. Doctor Robot didn't see a person in front of him. Kim was like a mannequin that he was required to inject once a month. No need to feel any empathy towards a mannequin.

We would find out later just how little empathy he had.

SPIES IN FLORIDA

YOU READ THAT CHAPTER TITLE and thought to yourself, "No way." Yes way. The Big Z hired private eyes to spy on Kim in Florida. When we discovered this we were astonished. We thought we had left all that behind. We had made a new life for ourselves. Kim wasn't better but she seemed to be stabilizing. Now all the bad memories and all of the old stressors came flooding back like a dam had burst. It was unbelievable. It was extremely disheartening. Kim cried for days. Her pain level shot back up to maximum agony.

First the spies came to the marina. They posed as tourists with cameras and photographed us on the boat. They watched us from public areas in plain view. We had no idea this was going on. Reports were going back to Big Z anytime Kim did anything that was perceived as physical. It didn't matter how small. Look, Kim is carrying a bag. Look, Kim is folding laundry. Let's send her back to work. She doesn't need all this expensive medical care. The expensive medical care was keeping her alive. Just maybe, it might improve her quality of life. Big Z cared for no such thoughts.

Kim's previously well-considered paranoia returned. Every strange car in the parking lot was an agent of Big Z. She was right again. They were out there. They were watching her.

We had gotten pretty comfortable with living on the boat. We decided to leave the marina to avoid the spies. This would be a huge step for us, especially for Kim. In a marina you have unlimited water supply and electricity. Away from the marina you have water holding tanks and a generator. Things would change. Life would be tougher. To get to shore we would use a dinghy. Kim had difficulty getting in and out of the dinghy. Life would become more spartan and less luxurious. We'd be roughing it, somewhat. Once again Kim said "I'm game." She's so awesome.

We needed to take baby steps. We left the marina but anchored close by, just off a public park. We'd get our sea legs, get used to living at anchor, then take off for parts unknown. We started making short trips to the coast to anchor among the barrier islands. We'd return to the park anchorage in order to resupply and keep appointments. We stretched ourselves a little longer each time, just getting acquainted with living away from the marina.

Big Z spied on us from the park when we were in town. They took pictures of Kim sitting on the back of the boat in her bathrobe. They filmed her riding in the dinghy. They filmed her walking to the truck. We didn't find this out until much later. If we'd known, we would have disappeared forever. We would have left town with no forwarding address and never come back.

Thinking back and realizing that we were being watched like that infuriates me. Their surveillance of us was an unbelievable violation of our privacy. You think Big Brother is watching? Big Z is watching, a lot. For all we knew, Big Z was watching us eat, sleep, read, hug and kiss. Their telephotos could probably see the title of the book in our hands.

We were zoo exhibits for who knows what kind of perverts. Even though we were unaware, at least at first, our lives were no longer ours alone. We were sharing it with Big Z. Did they have pictures of us showering too?

Kim was being a real trouper about living at anchor. She didn't mind the limited space or not being able to touch land. She wasn't exactly active. She would just sit and read or do crossword puzzles most of the time. I can't imagine it was very exciting for our voyeurs. As for going to land, I mostly did that by myself. I'd take the dinghy and get to the grocery store, or haul our trash. For appointments I'd gingerly help her off the swim platform into the dingy, then calmly drive us in to shore and help her out. I'd hold onto her until we got to solid ground, then she could walk on her own for a short distance.

It had to drive our spies crazy. They were conducting the most boring surveillance ever. Eventually they got tired of waiting for something to happen, so they took matters in to their own hands.

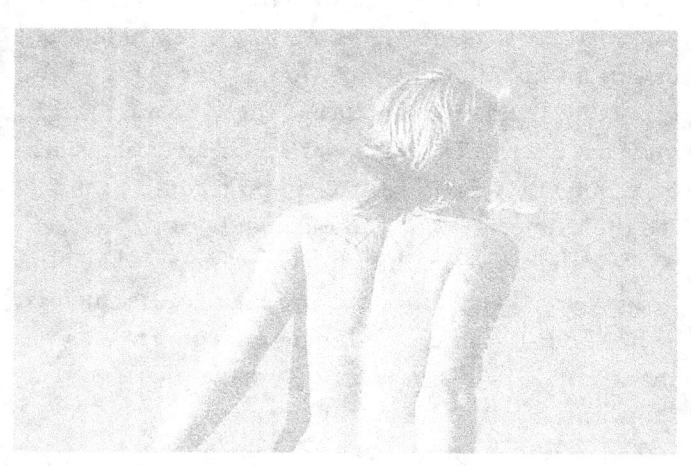

DOCTORED VIDEO

I DO NOT KNOW IF IT was the spies, someone at Big Z, or someone associated with The Dick, but videos were presented that were heavily edited. They managed to run enough tape, cut out everything that would hurt their case, and come up with several instances of Kim looking "normal."

They left out the footage of me lowering Kim into the dinghy. They left out the part where I lifted her out of the dinghy. They neglected to include her struggle up the dock, with one arm in mine and the other on the rail. They did show her walking in the parking lot. They did not show her stop to rest halfway through a fifty-yard walk.

In other instances they left out her sitting on the ground holding her leg, waiting out a spasm brought on by walking. They didn't include any of the dozen times she vomited into a bag or alongside the truck. They certainly didn't include the time she actually fell hard as we tried to board the dinghy. They just had several minutes of footage of her walking, on different days in different places. They just had Kim sitting upright in the dinghy as I drove on a calm day. It was all very boring yet appeared very normal. They managed to make Kim seem like a reasonably healthy person by omitting anything that showed otherwise. It was despicable.

The Bulldog called us with the alarming news. The Dick had filed on behalf of Big Z to terminate any future payment of medical expenses. As a matter of fact, payment for treatment or medication was suspended immediately, pending a new hearing. She had seen the videos and admitted that nothing seemed to be wrong in them. I had not seen the videos, and couldn't rebut them without seeing them. I was beside myself. I'd have to break the news to Kim, and I knew what it would do to her.

It went as I expected it would. Kim broke down. It hit her extremely hard. She sunk to the floor and sobbed. It would be weeks or months but soon we'd have to return to Delaware for Kim to be re-examined. We couldn't see the doctor, get injections, or fill prescriptions unless we paid for everything ourselves. Each medication was several thousand dollars for a thirty-day supply. The injections were many thousands as well. We'd be flat broke in a few months. Then what?

I was stunned. Once again, I just didn't know what to do or say. I wanted to hold Kim tight and tell her everything was going to be all right, but I wasn't sure I believed that myself. So I held her in silence while she sobbed. When she started to calm down she said, "What are we going to do?" All I could think of was to run. "Let's pull up anchor and run away for a while." It was late in the day to leave for our favorite anchorage on the coast, so I immediately prepared to get underway. I didn't give her time to think it over.

We pulled up anchor and made a run for it. All during our four-hour voyage the phone rang. Bulldog was on the job. Kim got mad instead of sad and handled the calls with a firm voice. She didn't quiver or sugarcoat her feelings. Our lawyer referred us to a state-run system that would cover meds until the hearing. If we won, then Big Z would have to foot the bill. If we lost, we wouldn't have to repay them. The pills would come by mail, with no further doctors' visits. Kim made arrangements for the meds to be shipped to a friend's house.

After multiple calls back and forth, Kim told Bulldog that we didn't want to be bothered for a few weeks. Don't call us, we'll call you. We were going off-grid for a while. If was after dark when we made the entrance to Pelican Bay. We had witnessed a beautiful sunset over the Gulf of Mexico an hour before. Once we got settled on our anchor, we sat quietly on the back of our boat. There was no traffic noise, no phone ringing, no sirens or really any noise at all. The gentle lapping of water on the hull was the only sound. We sat quietly. Occasionally Kim would breathe a deep sigh.

It was not an uncomfortable silence. It was welcomed. It was therapeutic. Running away may not be the best answer to life's problems, but right then it seemed like a wonderful solution. We would eventually deal with it, but the lawyers would have to wait.

That night Kim slept. Through the next morning she slept. She slept well into the afternoon. I checked to make sure she was breathing she slept so long. For several years she never slept more than a few hours at a time. Even that was fitful sleep. On this night she was a log. She wasn't tossing and turning. She was still. I didn't know if it was exhaustion from the most recent ordeal, or the fact that we were anchored in paradise.

The next few weeks were like a dream. I took Kim to the beach every day that she was up to it. We'd sit in our beach chairs and stare at the Gulf. We'd let the waves lull us into a peaceful bliss. Kim read books, continued to sleep late and even ate a little better. I started to venture off in the mornings while she slept. I did a lot of fishing. No offense to Kim, but it was nice to have a few hours to myself now and then. I was able to clear my head. I'd come back and we'd fix breakfast before going to the beach again. We watched the sunset together every night. Far from the city lights, we saw a million stars after dark.

When I sensed she was ready, I broached the subject of our eventual return to lawyers, drugs, and money. She hated the idea of going back to face another trying ordeal, but she said yes, let's get it over with.

We made the call to Bulldog. We'd have to fly in, and get a rental car, and a hotel would be provided. They would reimburse us for Kim's expenses, but not for mine. There was no way Kim could travel on her own. I demanded they cover my airfare and they relented.

She was to be examined by the same "independent" physician that saw her before the first hearing. Next would be a skills assessment test, lasting several hours. Both appointments were on the same day. Kim was expected to fly in the night before. She was to fly out the next day after two separate exams. I knew that was impossible. I'd work it out.

We both dreaded what was to come, but Kim was determined to be strong. She'd go and submit to their exams. She knew her disability was real. If she had to go through more pain to prove it, then so be it.

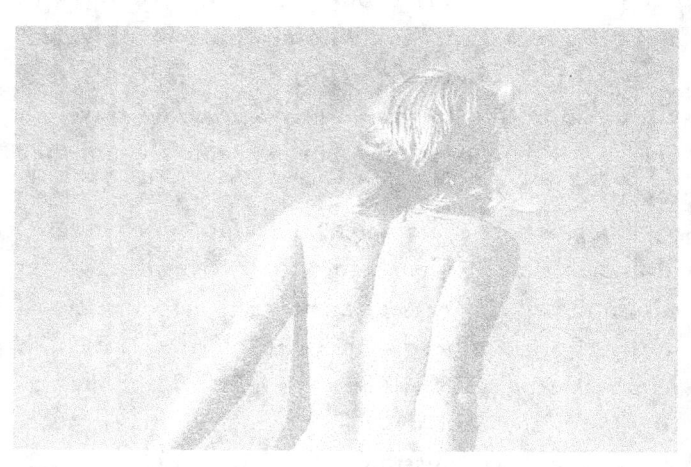

FALSE STATEMENTS

WE FLEW IN TO BALTIMORE after dark. It was a long walk to the rental car pickup so I borrowed a wheel chair for Kim. We drove over an hour to the ratty Radisson they had put us in. We knew we were being watched, or at least assumed we were. By the time we checked in Kim was pretty beat. The drive to the airport in Florida, the flight itself, the drive to the hotel, all this was ten times more activity than she was used to.

When I woke her the next morning her pain was pretty bad. This was going to be a long day. We nibbled on some cardboard muffins offered as a continental breakfast before leaving for the first appointment.

We didn't like this doctor the first time we saw him. It was obvious that he was a paid shill for the insurance company. He blundered badly during the workman's comp hearing and Bulldog made him look like a fool. He held that against us. His exam was worthless. He asked some questions and made gestures that signaled he didn't believe the answers.

He allowed us to waste a few minutes of his time, then went off to report how healthy Kim was to Big Z.

One appointment was out of the way but we didn't like how things were going. We had an hour to kill before the next one. Kim was uncomfortable and fidgety. We drove through a bad neighborhood looking for the next doctor. We found him in a rat-infested strip mall, next to a check cashing store and a pawn shop. I'm not making this up.

He took Kim into a room that was half gym and half workshop. He explained that Kim would be required to perform a variety of tasks of increasing difficulty. She could stop when she could no longer continue each task. I was not allowed to assist her at any time for any reason. He wouldn't let me touch her. When he gave her a break I took her arm to help her up and he scolded me.

He gave Kim a milk crate and told her to put it up on the table. She did. Then he added weight to the crate. He continued to add weight until she couldn't lift it. He made her walk backwards and crawl on the floor. He made her stand on one leg. She could do this with her good leg, but not on her little leg. Soon she began to break down.

She started to cry and couldn't complete the simplest tasks, things she could normally do. He asked her to climb a ladder. She refused. Her face was flushed and she was sweating. I tried to intervene and was again scolded. This was going horribly. Kim made only a half-hearted effort at the next few tasks and finally quit. She wasn't taking this anymore. It was humiliating her. Out the door we went.

We were supposed to return to the Radisson but we didn't. Instead we drove an hour south, keeping watch for a tail. When we were positive we weren't being followed, we got a nice hotel room for the night. We'd fly out the next day, after Kim got some rest. We still had a long way to go before we were safely aboard *Leap of Faith*.

We spoke with our lawyer and everything was set except for one thing. Robot Doctor was refusing to give a deposition. We had begged him several times but he always put us off. All we needed was for him to say that the treatments were medically necessary. Bulldog assured us that if he would put that in writing, we'd have no trouble. The fact that he was in a different state meant that he was not compelled to give the deposition by law. The fact that he had no compassion was another thing all together.

Bulldog also assured us that we would lose without a deposition from a treating doctor. Robot was the only doctor we had, and he was not willing to help. We returned to Florida with very low spirits. The entire trip had been a disaster. The gains Kim had made while sunning on the beach were all gone, and then some.

We hated lawyers and doctors more than ever. We tried to arrange a visit with our old friend the Witch Doctor. He assured us that he'd see Kim, give her an injection, and write the deposition. He said he would have the Wiccan arrange it.

Too much time passed with no word from the Wiccan. We called and called and got the runaround from a new girl in the office. At one point we actually thought we had an appointment; she just needed to confirm. The confirmation never came. We couldn't make the flight arrangements without it. We called again and left message after message. We had Bulldog call. We never did hear back from the Wiccan. We had given her our favorite sofa and she let us down. When we needed her she wasn't there for us.

We ran out of time, and a decision on Kim's fate was going to happen without any representation from a medical professional on her side. What we didn't know was that those two examiners from our horrible trip would make false statements. Having been showed the doctored video, they agreed to claim Kim was faking *before* ever examining her. The exams were a sham. Their minds were already made up, thanks to a healthy check from Big Z.

It was hopeless. We had lost. There would be no more medicine, no more injections, and no more care for Kim. I can't properly put into words just how dejected we were. Every time Kim had been beaten down, she had managed to get back up. I couldn't see how she would ever get up from this one. I feared for her. I feared she would give up. I feared for her heart and her soul. I feared for her life.

MOVING ON

WE HAD NO CHOICE BUT to just keep moving on. Kim had a fresh supply of meds. We figured out that the company providing them through the mail hadn't yet been notified that we no longer qualified for their assistance. We put in another order even though she already had three months' worth. When it came in we had almost a six-month supply.

We had no doctor's appointments to keep, no obligations. We really had no place to be and we certainly didn't want to anchor off that park again. It was time to leave. We loaded up the boat with all the food, booze, and supplies we could stow. We returned to our little piece of heaven in Pelican Bay with plans to stay for months.

It was actually quite a relief to be finished with the lawyers and the doctors. We lost, but we had no reason to fight anymore. All we had to worry about was our boat and each other. We still had money in the bank. We were going to drop out of society and not look back. We had no plan when it came to Kim's pills. It would be many months before she ran out. I realize it may seem irresponsible of us, not trying to find a way to continue her treatment. But we were beaten. We only wanted to sail off into the sunset. We only wanted a return to those few weeks when we were happy and all was right with our world. The rest of the world could go on without us. We wanted nothing to do with it.

We found our idyllic spot just the way we'd left it. Beautiful, peaceful, and well- protected. We set up our floating homestead just where we liked to be. It took a few weeks, but Kim started sleeping twelve hours or more each night. Over the past month, her weight loss had accelerated. She'd already become dangerously thin, but was now down to one hundred and five pounds. Remember, she's almost six feet tall. She was a walking warning against anorexia. Her ribs were all very visible. Her arms were twigs. Her hair was so thin I thought she might go bald soon. She took to wearing a ball cap to cover her hair. She was existing on yogurt and fruit snacks. Sometimes she would even throw up the yogurt.

We ignored all of that. We got back into the old routine. I'd let her sleep until noon while I went off fishing or exploring. We'd cook breakfast for lunch and head off for the beach. Over time, she began to take short walks on the beach. She developed an interest in collecting shells. If she couldn't walk the beach that day, I'd find a bunch of pretty shells for her.

One day we discovered Sand Dollar Beach. The tide was very low and a sandbar was exposed. Together we collected over a hundred sand dollars. We were like small children in our glee. What a treasure we had found. We began to live for simple pleasures. I never tired of taking my coffee with the dolphins at sunrise. We never missed a sunset together. Shells and sand dollars were like gold coins to us.

It was a very gradual process, but Kim was improving. Without the multitude of stresses that had hounded her the past four years, she began to find herself again. In tiny increments she was feeling stronger. The pain was ever-present, but her ability to get up and walk around, to enjoy the beach and our simple pleasures, was increasing.

One day on the beach she turned to me and said, "I'm going to cut back a little on the pills in order to preserve my supply." I offered that it was up to her. If she felt she could do it, then great. She immediately cut the Nucynta down from three times per day to twice a day. We noticed the difference immediately. At the eight hour mark, when she would normally take another pill, she would start to hurt. She'd be in rough shape for four hours until she took the next pill. She was taking them in the morning and at night before bed. So in the evenings she was in great pain.

That was when we discovered the pain-killing properties of rum. I'm not making this up either. When the pain would become too much to bear, we'd start doing shots of rum. After a few shots were tossed back, the pain was under control. Kim emphatically insisted that out of all the medications she had taken, rum worked the best to control her pain. We became rummies. Every night at six we would do a shot of rum. Every half hour after that we'd do another shot, until we fell asleep. It may have been six shots or it may have been eight. Kim and I both went to bed feeling no pain.

Since that time I've done some research, as I am prone to do. It turns out that rum has long been known to have health benefits, including lowering blood pressure and reducing stress. We were all about reducing stress.

Several studies have shown that moderate amounts of rum lower the risk of kidney disease, non-Hodgkin's lymphoma, and thyroid cancer. Longevity is often associated with drinking rum. A lower incidence of coronary disease may be a contributing factor. Anxiety reduction and a reduced risk factor for Alzheimer's and dementia have been cited as additional benefits of drinking rum. We most likely exceeded what would be considered moderate intake, but it certainly seemed to help.

Another med I forgot to mention was the muscle relaxer Baclofen. Eventually Kim dropped that dose from three times a day to twice a day. The original idea was to save them up so the total supply would last longer. The muscle relaxer was helping to prevent cramps and spasms in her leg. At first the spasms returned due to the lower dosage, but eventually they lessened. She was getting by with one less narcotic per day and one less muscle relaxer. She maintained this regimen for several more months. Eventually she was doing pretty well, even with the lower doses.

We were becoming sun worshippers and beach addicts. Our trips to the beach were as important as the meds for Kim. If the weather turned bad and we couldn't make it to the beach for a few days, Kim would suffer beach withdrawals. Her happy place was in that beach chair on Sand Dollar Beach. Her walks became more frequent and a little longer. She began to venture out into the Gulf to float in the warm water.

Keep in mind that this was a very gradual change. If I wasn't with her every minute of every day I wouldn't have seen it. We lived for the beach. The boat and our new life in this special place were doing wonders for her. Her aura changed, if that makes any sense. She smiled more. She laughed more. Her skin smoothed out with her new glowing tan. She was still weak and thin. She still battled pain every day. Her hair was hopeless, but her attitude was beginning to turn around. In moments when the pain wasn't unbearable, she could find some enjoyment. We were having logical and sensible conversations. Her mind was clearing up. We had no goals in life at all except her continued improvement. We had no bills to pay. No jobs to go to. We were beholden to no one. There were no doctors here, or lawyers. We had left that world behind and we existed for no one but each other.

We decided to broaden our horizons by taking trips to new places. We anchored on the inside of Sanibel Island near Ding Darling Wildlife Refuge. We were the only boat in sight. It was a scenic and peaceful place to be. When we needed a few supplies we took the boat to Fort Myers Beach. We didn't really want to go back where the spies lurked. No one knew where we were now. In Fort Myers Beach we could ride the dinghy right up to a grocery store. We could use the dinghy to visit waterfront restaurants. The beach was a short walk away, with plenty of places to stop and rest if needed.

With the boat resupplied, our trash disposed, of and our water tanks refilled, we returned to Pelican Bay with the knowledge we could last another month or more before revisiting civilization. We were becoming accustomed to our isolation. We enjoyed not being around other people. It was our own little world, just the two of us resting quietly in paradise. I felt that the rest and lack of negative stimulation was doing Kim some good. The changes were infinitesimal but they were there.

She had reduced her pill intake without major calamity. She didn't get worse as a result of fewer drugs. She could walk on her own most of the time, although if she overdid it she paid the consequences. She had abandoned the cane she once used for assistance. She was embarrassed by it, wouldn't use it in public places, and worked hard to walk with a normal gait when people she knew could see her. I started to have the slightest glimmer of optimism for her future. We still didn't know what we would do when the pills ran out. We didn't want to think about it. We wanted to stay lost in our endless summer just wasting away the days.

Little by little Kim started increasing how much she ate. She couldn't always keep it down, but she was making an effort to take in more calories. I had taken a picture of her on the beach in a bikini. She could see her bones all sticking out. She could count her ribs. She had a slightly distended belly like you see on starving children in Africa. She bottomed out at one hundred and two pounds on her six foot frame. Forty pounds had melted off her once sexy figure. She really did look like she was at death's door, but inside she was alive. Her eyes were clear and her mind was sharpening.

When she managed to actually gain a few pounds we were thrilled. Was this the turnaround we had hoped for? We agreed that the condition seemed to be stabilizing. We didn't have a doctor to consult with, but what good had they done? We became our own doctors. We decided what was good or bad for Kim without any professional input. If a certain food or activity made her feel better, we did more of that. If something made her worse, we eliminated that.

We were very attuned to her current physical condition and symptoms on a daily basis. Every morning I'd ask her how she was feeling. How's the leg? Did you sleep well? How's the stomach feeling? Are you hungry? She would give me honest feedback. We would decide together what steps to take next or what to do that day, based on how good or bad she felt. It was like she had her own personal nurse twenty-four hours a day. We did the give-and-take routine in the evenings as well. Did today's beach walk cause too much pain? Maybe tomorrow we'll just sit for a while instead of walking. We recalled how Doctor Drill Sergeant forbade her from walking in the sand. He said it would cause her problems and was not a good thing to do in her condition. She was proving him wrong, it seemed to us.

Her dark tan had erased the blotches and streaks in her skin. Even though she was weak and skinny, she now had a healthier glow. I think this helped her self- confidence some. No woman wants to have unsightly blotches and weird streaks in her skin. She was now wearing a ball cap every day, and I told her I always liked chicks in ball caps. At first she wore mine, but eventually we got her very own, more girlie, caps.

We were adjusting to her limitations. Apart from the pain we were enjoying this life. It felt so good to be away from the doctors and the stress. Kim abandoned the message board with other RSD sufferers. She said they were all so negative, and everyone had a sad story to tell. No one was finding relief or reporting on a new treatment effort that was actually helping them. We also abandoned the idea of going to Tampa for the ketamine treatments. A hospital was the last place Kim wanted to be, surrounded by doctors sticking her with needles. We saw logic in continuing what we were doing, whether it was right or wrong. It seemed to be working for her. The progress wasn't much, but it was a step in the right direction.

Kim gained approximately one pound per month until she was up to one fifteen. Her ribs were less pronounced and she was feeling stronger. We had made a few more boat trips along the west coast of Florida and were both more at ease with the handling of the boat and navigation. We decided to go on an extended trip. Again, we had no place to be. We could go anywhere we wanted.

In May of 2012, almost four years after her injury, we turned *Leap of Faith* south and headed for the Keys. We left Fort Myers Beach for Marco Island and enjoyed our very first successful offshore passage. The water was calm that day, and very blue. Kim reported no ill effects during the six-hour trip. We pulled up anchor the very next day and aimed our bow at the Everglades. Ten hours later we anchored in a protected cove just as a storm blew up. It continued to storm for several more days. We had no cell phone reception or Internet service. There was no place to get off the boat and onto land among the swampy mangrove-covered islands. The mosquitoes were outrageous. We holed up inside the boat for six days. Kim was none too happy.

On day seven she pronounced that we were leaving no matter what. "Get me the hell out of here," she said. "I don't care if we never make it to the Keys but I can't stay here another day." We pulled anchor before first light and poked our nose out into the Gulf. It was going to be rough, but it was doable. We crossed Florida Bay in the roughest seas we had ever experienced at the time. Kim was tense at first. I worried that the rolling of the boat would set off her pain. She settled in the first mate's chair and played games on her iPad, ignoring the tossing motion of our vessel. It wasn't exactly a fun crossing, but we finally made it to Marathon and Boot Key Harbor.

It had been a long day for both of us and Kim was worn out. We didn't go out for dinner or explore the town or do anything at all. I spent a few days walking to the grocery store and refilling the liquor cabinet while she rested. We hopped down to Bahia Honda eventually, then a place called Saddlebunch Key. Our last stop was to be Key West.

Key West is the end of the road and a popular place for misfits to hide. We decided we'd fit right in. If society's rejects congregated here, we figured our rejection of society earned us a spot at the bar. The atmosphere here is unique in America. The Conch Republic is like a country of its own. Everyone should visit at least once, but it turned out to be not for us.

We had to anchor pretty far away which made for long, bumpy dinghy rides. The climb onto the dinghy dock proved difficult for Kim. She would get on her hands and knees and literally crawl onto the dock. Before we ever set foot on land she was up a bit up on the pain level scale. The first day we only visited one establishment, because it was so close by. In the following days we managed to walk Duval Street. We could stop and sit at a bar anytime Kim needed to get off her feet, which meant our daily bar tab total was pretty high.

We did some tourist stuff and some not so touristy stuff. One late afternoon we found ourselves at Mallory Square in time for the daily sunset celebration. We couldn't miss it. It was an unforgettable time, but when it was over Kim was incapable of walking any further. We were far from our dinghy so I hailed us a pedicab. For fifteen bucks we got a nighttime ride back up Duval and over to the waterfront.

One day we attempted to make it to the Southernmost Point. Didn't happen. Kim collapsed on Duvall Street near Willy T's. I sat her at a table and got her some food and a cold drink. We lounged away the afternoon just allowing her to rest there. That pretty much made up my mind that it was time to leave.

The walking was too much. The noise and the excitement were too much. The crowds of people we were definitely not used to. It was time to pull up anchor and head north.

The trip north was uneventful, and things went smoothly. We made it back to Fort Myers Beach in time for our anniversary. While Kim slept one morning, I snuck into town to find something to give her. I stumbled across a medallion made of silver from the shipwreck *Atocha*. She was so surprised and happy with it. (We had quit giving each other gifts when we left our old lives behind, in order to save money.) She wore it that night when we went out to dinner. We listened to tropical music waterside and enjoyed a lovely anniversary together.

After once again resupplying in Fort Myers Beach, it was back home to Pelican Bay. Yes, we now considered this our home, and it was good to be back. Kim had survived a major excursion. She was emboldened. She suffered some setbacks along the way but was glad to have made the journey. It was a real turning point in her recovery. She was going to make it.

We didn't know if she would ever return to her former self, but she wasn't going to die. She was going to be okay.

DOPE

Now that we were back in familiar surroundings, we went back to our old routine. We didn't get much beach time on our trip to the Keys. It was nice to feel the sand between our toes again. By now we were convinced that the simple act of sitting on the beach was beneficial to Kim. Not only was the ocean helping her physically recover, it was healing her soul. I have to admit, it was doing wonders for mine too.

Out of nowhere, on the beach one day, Kim said, "I feel good." The walks had grown longer and more frequent. We explored the islands more. She was definitely getting better. She announced that she would cut back on the Marinol. When she told me that, I got the brilliant idea that smoking pot might be better than taking synthetic marijuana. I've read lots of stories from cancer patients who reported all sorts of benefits from smoking weed. I even knew one personally. We also had several friends who smoked recreationally. We decided to look into the matter further.

In the meantime, she took one less Marinol pill per day. We could see no ill effects due to the lesser dosage. Her appetite did not decrease, and her nausea did not get worse.

In order to secure some marijuana, though, we'd have to return to the town that used to have spies. Coincidentally, some friends of ours had just bought a house that we could get our boat up to. We could sneak into town and not be seen. Then came the matter of how to approach our smoking friends to ask to buy some pot. I had no idea how this worked. I didn't know what it cost or how much to buy. Thankfully, our kind friends guided us through and we were soon the proud owners of a little bag of weed.

We didn't really know what to do with it once we had it, but we'd figure something out once we got away from town again. On the boat back in Pelican Bay I fashioned a pipe out of some brass fittings and we were ready. I didn't want to smoke any of it. Kim insisted that she didn't want to do it by herself. That first night we both smoked just a little bit. I can't say I enjoyed it. It was pleasant enough, but just not my cup of tea. After that Kim was on her own.

She abandoned the Marinol altogether and went strictly with the real thing. A couple times per day was doing the trick. She started eating better. She had less nausea. Now, I'd never been a big fan of marijuana. It just didn't appeal to me. The medical marijuana issue never affected me one way or the other. Now it was having a direct effect on me, or at least my wife. It helped her. I've seen it help others. I'm now a believer. There is no doubt in my mind that marijuana can help people who are suffering.

Kim had completely eliminated one of the drugs she was previously prescribed. She had reduced her intake of the others by one-third. Not only was she not worse off, she was getting better. The trend was undeniable. She then quit taking the anti-nausea pill. There was no longer a need for it. She still had a hefty supply of Marinol and the anti-nausea pills, but she never went back to them. They were out of her life forever.

She was really proud of herself. She began to hate the pills she was still taking. She told me that one day she was going to stop and never take pills again. Her confidence and optimism were improving daily. She had that goal to be pill-free and she was certain she could do it. The uplift in her spirit seemed to translate into more improvements in her physical condition. She would occasionally have a great day when she seemed to be perfectly normal. Bad weather or too much activity would put her back down again, but she was obviously on the upswing.

I was happy for a number of reasons. My wife was getting well again. She had suffered so much over the past five years. To see her smile and laugh just lifted me up. To walk with her on the beach of Cayo Costa, hand in hand, was a blessing from God. I also felt vindicated about my choices. Quitting my job and living on a boat was turning out to be a very good thing. Running away after we lost the case turned out to be a good thing. You never know for sure where your choices are going to take you in life. I had hoped that mine would be helpful to Kim, but I could never guarantee it. Now it looked like I did the right thing, and I didn't do it by myself. Kim was making those same choices right along with me. At any time she had the freedom to back out. She forced me to promise her that, when we left our old life. If she wanted off the boat and back on land, then I had to respect her wishes. Instead she had taken to the boat life quite well. She wouldn't dream of returning to a land based life.

We took a huge leap of faith and it looked more and more certain that it would work out for the best. We owe everything to taking that leap.

Eventually Kim would give up smoking dope. She improved so much that she didn't need it anymore. It still felt wrong to her; after all, it was illegal. We felt like criminals buying it and hiding it. It seemed so silly to have to sneak around in order to get it. Generally we are law-abiding types. To be marked a criminal for smoking a natural substance that helps to ease your pain now seems very wrong to us. We never really thought about it before. We know different now.

Kim never did take another Marinol pill after quitting marijuana. She did continue to drink rum.

NEW ADVENTURES

WE SUFFERED A MINOR SETBACK when Kim reduced her medications once again. She was now taking just one Nucynta and one Baclofen each morning. She wasn't making it through the day without experiencing pain and leg cramps. The smallest activity would spike her pain. Even the running of the boat's engine would cause her discomfort.

We laid low for a while and she fought off the urge to take more medicine. She simply refused to resort to the pills when things got bad. I felt bad for her, but I was proud of her new found determination. She was on a mission to rid herself of drugs. Each time she had managed to take less, her condition had improved. She was convinced that if she could get off the pills altogether, she would have beaten RSD.

Over time she adjusted to the lower doses. She was well enough to start mixing with society in small doses. Using our friends' dock, we started visiting the old spy town to listen to our favorite musicians or meet up for drinks. Most of the people in that little community never knew the extent of Kim's illness. Some knew that "something" was wrong, but not to what extent or exactly was the cause was.

Her reintroduction to society really brought her out of her shell. We went to a party and she danced. Not really dancing; more standing in one place and shaking around a bit. She laughed and smiled and had a great time. There was no doubt she had turned it around.

We even took more boat trips, exploring places like Long Boat Key and Anna Maria Island. She was able to enjoy the new sights. We walked new beaches and had happy hour on new sand bars. We walked the paths at De Soto Park and explored Bradenton Beach. This was a whole new life for us. We weren't hidden away in a quiet little cove with no other people around. We were seeing new places, having new adventures.

We did this in whatever small doses Kim could withstand. Any time she felt she needed to, we would retreat to the boat and be by ourselves. We always returned to Pelican Bay whenever we needed to feel at home.

On these explorations Kim transformed from a crippled recluse, to a sporty adventurer. She regained almost all the weight she had lost. She had less muscle tone than when she was well, but she looked good. I took her to an expensive salon to have her hair looked at. She spent a day and hundreds of dollars having it treated with all sorts of potions. It helped give her some body and she started a Moroccan oil treatment that continued to improve the thickness. Her hair came almost back to normal. She still wore ball caps but not as often.

As much as the solitude and peace of the beach helped her early on, these new trails we were blazing were helping her now. She was no longer embarrassed to be seen in public. She got bolder, doing new things and going new places. We could go longer and harder than ever before. Dinghy rides didn't kill her. Her increasing ability to withstand more and more physical activity was allowing us to expand the scope of our travels. We could better enjoy the sights and sounds of new places without worrying that she would break down.

My lovely wife was back. We still had to make allowances from time to time, but those times were becoming rare. Bad weather still had a negative effect on her. We noticed a correlation between a low barometer and increased pain. Over exertion was still something we had to guard against. She felt better and she wanted to do more and more. Sometimes it was too much.

We even started to make love again. Not as often as we once did, but it was nice when it happened. We couldn't be any closer as a couple. She started to seek out more hugging and touching. She said she just needed to be close to me. We had been through a lot together, and come out of it with our marriage intact.

I know that she feels like she couldn't have done it without me. I also know that I'd be nothing without her. We managed to survive together. We will stay together no matter what the future brings.

THE LAST OF
THE DRUGS

WE WERE ENJOYING SOME DOWN time in Pelican Bay, relaxing after our latest adventure. Kim was feeling particularly well. We were extremely happy. We enjoyed our sunsets and our nightly shots of rum. We made love on the bow of our boat with no one in sight. Life couldn't get any better for us.

We thanked our lucky stars that somehow it had all managed to work out. I looked out on the ocean, and I wondered how we ever came this far. I had escaped corporate politics and a job I hated. I was once the boss of many, became a caregiver for a stricken wife, and ended up a carefree beachcomber. Kim had gone from being a vibrant host to celebrities, to a victim of a strange disease, and ended up a happy boat bum.

There was one last piece of the puzzle that Kim was absolutely determined to fit into place. She had been taking just one muscle relaxer and one painkiller for many months. Now she wanted to stop. Now was the time, she said. "I'm not taking any more pills. I'm quitting today and I'll never take another pill again."

That day she took no pills. Twenty-four hours later she was deathly ill. She had horrible stomach cramps. She was vomiting like the girl in "The Exorcist." She had bad diarrhea. Her entire body was racked with spasms and cramps. She was sweating, crying and in great distress. We were hours away from help.

As I knelt beside her, she gritted her teeth and said, "I'm not taking any more pills." She was going through withdrawal. The one narcotic pill per day had been just enough to keep that from happening. Now she had a choice, just like a junkie. Take the drug and feel better, or face days of agony. Neither of us had considered the possibility that she would face anything like this. She had done so well cutting back. On the other hand, her body had been accustomed to getting its daily fix for the last five years. It was punishing her with a vengeance.

This was Kim's moment of truth. All that she had been through, all the pain and all the loss boiled down to this moment. She had fought and fought until I was sure she couldn't fight anymore. She had won. She had beaten it, but here she was with one more battle to fight. I was by her side, but I was helpless to intervene. I couldn't fix this. I couldn't decide for her. She had to face this demon herself.

She struggled to sit up in bed as I brought her a glass of water. With tears streaming down her face she took my hand and said, "I'm not taking anymore pills. I won't do it." I think I would have taken a pill if I were in her shoes. She's the strong one. She is only better today through the force of her will. There was no one to see her incredible courage but me. I wanted to shout out, "Do you see this woman's strength?" As much as I was concerned for her, I couldn't have been more proud.

I took a minute to assess our situation. I decided we needed to get to civilization. When I told her I was pulling up anchor and heading to town, she said she did not want to see a doctor. I convinced her we needed to get her closer to one just in case. As I left her room she yelled after me. "I'm not taking any damn pills!"

The friends with the dock allowed us to tie up. They even allowed us to use their house, as they were away on business. I took Kim in and laid her down on the bed. She was pampered with air conditioning and a hot shower. She put cool dishcloths on her forehead. She lay in the dark room and stood up to the demon. She fought him off. At first he kept coming back for more, but he eventually tired. She outlasted him. For three days she kept up the battle. On day four she emerged victorious. She was once again weak and hungry, but she was once again a winner.

While she regained her strength she had a sense that her blood pressure was really high. This continued even after the effects of withdrawal had worn off. It was serious enough that she relented and agreed to see a doctor. They were appalled that she had gone cold turkey without medical supervision. Her pressure was indeed very high. She didn't go into the whole discussion about hating doctors with them. She did accept a prescription for blood pressure medication. She was going to have to take a pill after all. Eventually her pressure would come under control, but she is still reliant on this particular medication to this day. She has attempted to stop taking it too, but each time her pressure spikes almost immediately. She has come to terms with this and is resigned to continue taking it for the foreseeable future.

At least it's not a narcotic. The types of codeine and morphine that she had been on are every bit as powerful as heroin. They are highly addictive. They are also prescribed like candy to anyone with a back ache. Be very careful if you or a loved one is ever prescribed these drugs. You don't want to go through what Kim has gone through.

All of Kim's multiple doctors were more than happy to continue to prescribe these drugs to Kim regardless of the dangers or side effects. Only one privately owned pharmacy questioned her, out of the dozens we used.

Like I said earlier, I don't know if I would have had the same willpower that she had. It would have been so much easier for her to just take another pill. She did not. She is probably alive today because of her sheer willpower. The doctors didn't cure her. The pain management specialist couldn't control her pain. The insurance company skirted the law in order to get rid of her. It turns out that losing coverage for her treatment and medications was the best thing that ever happened to us.

She wasn't healed by modern medicine. She was healed by the sea. The beach cured her. The solitude and the serenity made her well. The absence of stress was a medicine in itself. The sounds of nature facilitated her revival. The breath of dolphins urged her to go on.

The doctors did nothing. The pills did nothing. The insurance company did nothing.

Modern medicine was killing my wife. She cured herself.

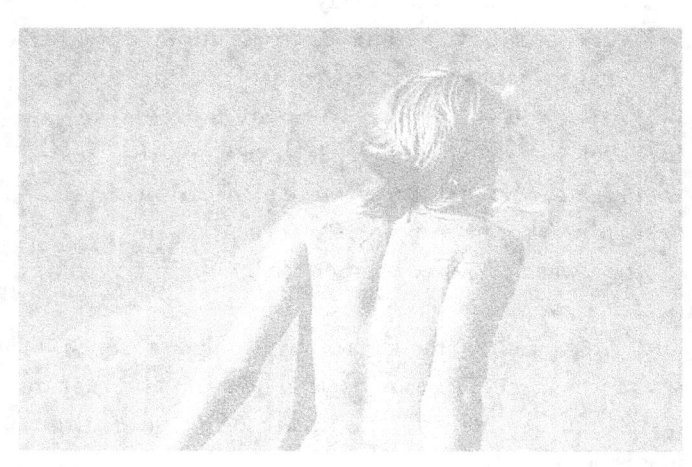

RUNNING LOW
ON MONEY

KIM WAS WELL ON HER way to recovery and we were living life in a dream. We had tropical beaches to lie on. We had an endless supply of life-enhancing sunshine. We played with the dolphins and manatees. Stress was almost completely non-existent for us now.

We had grown so very comfortable living out among the barrier islands that we never wanted it to end. We had one last little problem. After years with no income we were dangerously low on funds. The savings had dwindled away. We tried to avoid thinking about it for a time, but soon enough we'd have to seek a means of financial support.

Over the past six months I had written a book. It was in rough manuscript form, jotted down on a series of yellow legal pads. I needed to get it typed into a Word document and I needed a reliable Internet connection to finalize things with the publisher. We had no choice but to return to civilization in order to get the book published. I knew it was a long shot but I was determined to see it through.

While discussing our lack of funds one evening over cocktails, Kim insisted that she would be the one to get a job. She told me she would be happy to wait tables or take whatever employment she could find. She said she really wanted to go back to work. She felt that good. I couldn't let her work while I lounged, so it appeared we would both be looking for a job.

We made our preparations and took *Leap of Faith* up Charlotte Harbor to the beautiful town of Punta Gorda, Florida. We took a mooring ball off Laishley Park Marina in order to get rid of our trash, take long hot showers, and do our laundry. Laishley Park is a fine marina, which previously had not allowed slip holders to live aboard their boats. We noticed some folks who appeared to be doing just that. We asked the dock master about this, and he told us the rules had changed. He handed us a rate sheet and we returned to the boat to think things over.

That night we weighed to pros and cons of renting a slip in a marina. The cost was the first concern, but it would sure be nice to have constant electricity and hot water. If we were commuting back and forth to jobs, bad weather would make dinghy rides to shore very difficult. We decided to sign on for six months in the marina. Getting jobs was now an urgent priority. Paying slip rent would empty our savings in rapid fashion.

I went to the public library and made a resume for Kim. Her work history was pretty impressive, but the five year gap in employment looked suspicious. We agreed that she wouldn't mention it unless asked. She immediately applied at a dozen restaurants within walking distance of the waterfront. When prospective employers commented on the missing five years, she told them we'd been out cruising on our boat all that time. This was the truth, just not the entire truth.

It was early in the season in this resort town. Some establishments were interested in Kim, but told her they wouldn't hire for another month. I worked desperately to polish my hand-scribbled manuscript into something ready to print. Meanwhile we completely ran out of cash. Kim took a one-night job for cash. We used the forty bucks she earned to buy a few groceries. Things started to look bleak for us in the money department.

When I finally submitted my manuscript, I turned to job-seeking. I quickly picked up a part-time job in the marina. Kim continued to pound the pavement, handing out a resume to anyone who would accept it. My first few small paychecks quickly evaporated until the marina gave me extra hours. Kim's search wasn't going well at all.

The day arrived for my first book to go live at Amazon and Barnes & Noble. Much to our surprise, it was a big success. *Leap of Faith: Quit Your Job and Live on a Boat* climbed the rankings and garnered excellent reviews. It was a heady time for us, but the royalties would be slow in coming. I had a bestseller on my hands, but I continued to clean bathrooms and pick up trash at the marina. Kim finally landed a job but it didn't last long. She had trouble carrying heavy trays and keeping up with the fast pace. A second job didn't pan out either.

On my days off I banged away at my laptop, furiously pumping out a second book. I tirelessly promoted the first one and started blogging and developing a brand for myself using social media. Kim eventually found a job that fit. She brought home steady cash from her tips and we could eat again. Her return to the workforce was not an easy one. She came home dead tired with an assortment of aches and pains. At times she felt she couldn't go on. The old pain she experienced with RSD would try to creep back in. She maintained her steadfast refusal to resort to painkillers again.

I self-published a second book and it was an overnight sensation. We were amazed as *Poop, Booze, and Bikinis* rose to number one in Boating within twenty-four hours after its release. I started getting requests for interviews from web sites and radio stations. Royalties from the first book started to arrive. Things were looking up.

Kim was hanging in there at her job, but I could tell she wasn't happy with it. She had emerged victorious from her long battle with pain, but those five lost years had taken a toll on her body. She was offered a less physical position, as a boat rental agent right here in the marina. She accepted immediately.

Our bank account rose to a more comfortable level and we breathed a sigh of relief. Our financial future looks bright as royalties for two books start to pour in. We've adapted to life in the marina, but the islands call. We are both still working with the goal of replenishing the cruising kitty and once again living our dream.

Kim has taken back her life. She once was lost but now she's found. Both of us have a new found appreciation for the freedom we have experienced. The ordeal has strengthened us both. Our marriage couldn't be any stronger. We couldn't be any happier. Life is good today.

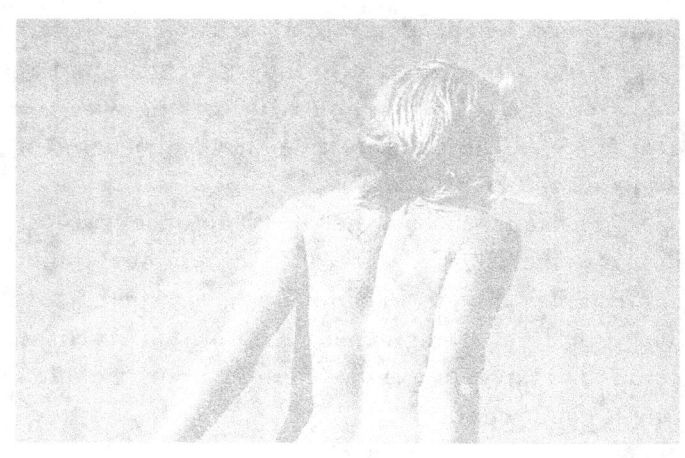

AUTHOR'S THOUGHTS

SOMETHING STRANGE HAPPENED TO ME while writing this book. The words came into my mind faster than I could type them. I wrote five thousand words every time I sat down at my laptop. The story consumed me. When I wasn't actually writing, it controlled my thoughts.

Kim read along as I worked. She had to relive some things she had forgotten purposefully. She cried from time to time, but urged me to continue. It was a cathartic experience for us both. When I finished, she told me that she felt free again. Telling her story was the final episode in her long struggle with pain. She could now put all those bad memories behind her. We hadn't given much thought to the future but now we could make plans. We could dream big again and maybe even take another leap of faith.

The ultimate goal of this work is to give hope to other sufferers. There were many times when Kim had no reason to hope for a better future. She was stuck in a seemingly endless cycle of pain. Somehow, she found a way out. We are not advocating that everyone dealing with chronic pain quit their job and live on a boat. That was our choice and it worked for us, but everyone has a different idea of what a stress-free environment would entail. We decided that eliminating stress was the best thing we could do for Kim. There was an absolute direct correlation between outside stress and her pain level. We also agreed all the stimulus in today's world only serves to increase one's stress. TV, cell phones, traffic noise, and the like bombard the senses twenty-four hours a day. We found peace in the lack of stimulus.

We are attempting to question how pain management is practiced in today's healthcare system. RSD/CRPS is a condition that is very poorly understood. Treatments for RSD and other forms of chronic pain are widely varied and controversial. Often the symptoms are treated and not the patient as a whole. In Kim's case, the treatments only made matters worse and few would listen to her complaints.

That person who carries a sometimes invisible burden of pain is often poorly understood too. "You don't look like you're hurt," is a common phrase heard by those with rare disorders. Doctors prescribe lethal doses of narcotics without a minutes care for the side effects. Nurses treat patients as if they were only drug seekers and not a living, breathing human being.

Most of the health care professionals that treated Kim over the years were either incompetent or uncaring. Of the five pain management specialists we saw, only the Witch Doctor seemed to really care about her well-being as a person. A twenty percent satisfaction rate doesn't speak well for the industry of pain management.

Dr. Quack and Dr. Senile had no business practicing medicine in any form. Christian Doctor put his petty grievance with the Witch Doctor over Kim's best interests. Dr. Drill Sergeant was a pawn of the insurance company. His only goal was to return Kim to the workplace and save Big Z some money. The same can be said for the patient advocate. Robot Doctor was an emotionless automaton who couldn't care less if Kim lost too much weight, vomited dozens of times daily and lost all of her hair. Writing a deposition to save her insurance coverage was too much of an imposition for him.

None of these highly educated professionals were able to offer anything to improve Kim's quality of life. We are fairly certain that they worsened her condition. We've all been ingrained to trust in the wisdom of our doctor. They are the expert. We learned that such trust is often misplaced. They don't always know what they are doing and no one is questioning them.

We also learned that some so-called physicians will say anything you want them to under oath, for a fee. The practice of insurance companies hiring any paid expert to testify against claimants is ridiculous. What's he going to do? Help Kim's cause? He's being paid to twist the truth or outright lie in order to protect the interests of the insurance company. I guess he's forgotten the Hippocratic oath.

Here are a few questions to think about. How much is the drug manufacturer paying you to prescribe a certain painkiller? How much kickback are you receiving per referral to a certain specialist? Is every care decision you make based on the patient's best interest, or your financial gain?

I don't mean to lump every health care professional together. I'm certain there are many wonderful doctors and nurses throughout our system. I'd say the same for school teachers, even though we know there are many teachers who shouldn't be in control of your child's education.

That brings me to the drug companies, or Big Pharma as people like to say. Why are drugs so expensive? Marinol is over fifteen hundred dollars for a 30-day supply. Most of the narcotics Kim took were just as expensive. Her monthly drug cache was worth approximately three thousand dollars. I understand that research, development, and testing are expensive endeavors. I also think they charge so much because they can. When most Americans have health insurance, they don't question costs. We learned that without health insurance, most doctors will charge you less for office visits. Full health insurance coverage for any petty issue is what drives costs in healthcare, in my opinion. Today everyone goes to the doctor for a simple cold. I also wonder how advertising affects cost. Do we really need to see the endless chain of drug commercials? Shouldn't those be directed at doctors and not patients? Don't get me wrong; I'm not against profits. I am against profits over people.

Let's discuss the legalization of medical marijuana. Who thinks that it's the drug companies keeping marijuana from being legalized? There have been hundreds of studies proving many useful benefits of marijuana. It's long been known that it helps glaucoma and cancer patients. Recent studies suggest that it may even cure certain types of cancer, not just treat the symptoms or side effects of chemo and radiation.

As I mentioned earlier, we never gave this topic much thought. After witnessing its positive properties I'm a believer and a brand new convert to the legalization cause. The evidence mounts daily in favor of approving marijuana for all types of patients. Withholding available relief to the sick and dying is unacceptable.

There are a lot of bad jokes about lawyers. Most of them are true. This profession is rife with greedy bastards who think nothing of the harm they cause. The Dick in this story was the epitome of the slime-balls portrayed in the jokes. He not only defended his client, he attacked Kim in a heartless manner. She has a lot of forgiveness in her heart, but not enough to let him off the hook for the way he treated her. How does such a person sleep at night? How does one gather the nerve to harass someone so obviously in pain? How does one justify hiring spies to stake out a person's home? How does one justify doctoring video in order to support your false claim? How does one sleep after paying off a witness to lie on the stand?

Our lawyer was on our side because we would eventually pay her. How would she react if she were in The Dick's shoes? She did a good job for us in the original hearing; for that she got to keep a third of Kim's meager award. (We knew that going in.)

Finally I ask, what was the responsibility of Kim's employer? During her protracted battle with the insurance company Dover Downs never once intervened or checked on her well-being. They did avail upon her to testify on their behalf in a sexual harassment case. An incident occurred while she was still employed and they summoned her to help their case, long after she had been terminated. They won that case, in part due to Kim's testimony. Could they have told the insurance company to back off? Should they have?

As a dedicated employee until her accident, she deserved, I feel, a lot more respect. She didn't hurt her back when no one was looking. It was her own boss who was responsible for her injuries. Delaware law says that you can't sue for a workplace injury unless you can prove negligence. No lawyer was willing to take on Dover Downs on these grounds.

The whole system is in chaos. Lawyers, doctors, and insurance companies coexist in some strange incestuous relationship that feeds on itself. They supply each other with business and scratch each other's backs to keep the gravy train rolling along. The victim is their last concern in a lot of cases. Before now I never railed against "The System," but seeing how it chewed Kim up and spat her out has changed my attitude.

Only through her extreme courage was she able to survive. Can you imagine what it took for her to agree to risk everything and go live on a boat? Taking that leap of faith was an incredibly brave thing for her to do. She had no guarantees. We didn't even dream that it would work out so well in the long run. She had been let down by The System. All of the doctors and lawyers and insurance companies failed her. She had her trust in me and her faith. She never lost either. Amid the chaos she was able to dream. She's a survivor of the highest degree. She took what threatened to destroy her and came out thriving.

Now she hopes that the questions her case asks can someday be answered. She wants to highlight the deficiencies in our treatment of chronic pain. She wants to propose that there is another way. She wishes to raise awareness of all these topics. Most of all she hopes that someone out there will be inspired to carry on. If her story can give hope to someone who is about to give up, it will all be worthwhile. If someone can't stand the pain any longer, but understands that Kim made it out, this book will be a success.

If only a handful of people read it, but those that do are able to continue their fight, then every word will be worth it. RSD doesn't have to be forever. It's real and it's painful and it's debilitating, but it can be defeated.

Let Kim be your guiding light.

AFTERWORD

BY KIM ROBINSON

I've cried more during the writing of this book than I have in years. My tears weren't due to sadness or pain, but from the awe I felt due to my husband's writing such a touching story about me. At first I didn't want the book to be written. I don't seek the limelight. As Ed said, we spent much of our time isolated from the outside world. The last thing I needed was any measure of fame.

But then as the book took shape I realized that it may be of some help to others who are now going through what I have been through. People with RSD/ CRPS, Fibromyalgia, etc. don't know where to turn. It often seems that there is no way out. They feel destined to live out their days in pain and suffering. Their loved ones seldom understand exactly what they are going through.

I can only say that I was lost. The horrible pain left me wanting to die. Some days I wished for death. It would be better than the way I was living. I was letting my children down at the most important time in their life. They needed me in ways that I just couldn't give. My most important job had always been as a mother.

Now I missed sporting events, retold the same stories over and over, and couldn't be there for them.

Then I had a choice. I could give in to the pain and let it control my life, or I could choose my children and my husband. I turned to prayer. I prayed a lot, not just for relief from the pain, but for my family. I took inspiration from my grandfather, who watched over me. I handed over my burdens to Jesus. In the end my prayers were answered. I was not destined to live out my life in pain and suffering.

All you victims of chronic pain need to know that. There is a way out. It may not be the same path that we traveled, but there is hope for you.

Ed described the various doctors quite accurately. At first I believed in them. I truly assumed they had my best interests at heart. Soon enough I began to lose faith in them. My voice wasn't being heard. Their methods were not helping. I hated being perceived as a druggie. The scrutiny I underwent on a daily basis was humiliating. The medical profession failed me. We had to find our own way.

My condition improved incrementally each time professional care was reduced. I finally began to heal when there was no medical treatment at all. I came to believe that natural forces within me, along with the sun and the serenity, would make me whole.

As for our escape, I was scared. I was deep inside my bubble of pain and about to leave all safety behind. I trusted my entire life to my husband. I knew that he would do his best to take care of me. His care is what saved me. He was fantastic. Our life on the boat gave me meaning. It gave me a safety net to relax in. It gave me time to heal. Relaxing in the sunshine with my husband was the best therapy I ever received.

Both of my children have grown up and decided to serve in the United States Marine Corps. I know that they are securely on their way and that they are content with their choice. Ed's daughter is happy with her spouse and two lovely children. Our children's success has eased my fears, which has eased my anxiety and truly eased my pain.

Ed talked about all the drugs and the bad effects they had on me. I don't remember a lot of it. I hope that he can forget any hurt that I caused him. I love him so much I'd never want to cause him even the slightest pain. He has been my rock throughout this journey. He is the strongest, most patient man I've ever met. He is also the kindest. He has earned my faith in him a thousand times over. On my darkest days, I could think to myself, "Ed will take care of me." He never let me down like all of those doctors did.

Since I've been off the meds I've gotten my life back. I'm stronger now. Still skinny but I'm thirty pounds heavier. I am more physical, can remember conversations and I don't look like a cripple. I am more comfortable in public and am much happier. I am more in love with my husband than I've ever been.

I can't properly express how grateful I am to Ed for helping me get well, and for writing this story. I'm also grateful that he didn't chase me around with pink elephants when I was high on ketamine. I love you with all of my heart.

"I'll be there, till the light dies in your eyes."

I also wish to give thanks to God. Somehow he saw fit to deliver me from evil.

Thanks to Jess and Daniel, my two Marines, for bearing with me when I was down, and for turning into fine young adults. You are both more than any mother could hope for.

Fondest thanks to Joseph V. Murphy, USMC. Granddad you will always be my hero. He always said to me, "I once cried because I had no shoes, until I met the man with no feet."

Thanks to my stepfather Jay, who was always more of a real father to me than that other guy. You didn't have to accept me as your own, but you always did.

I have to also thank all of my friends both past and present. Your acceptance of me really means a lot.

Of all of the doctors I had the displeasure of seeing, only one seemed to really care about me. Singing "Mrs. Robinson" to me while sticking a needle in my spine was a special touch. You'll always be my favorite Witch Doctor.

If you enjoyed this book, please write a review at Amazon.com.

ACKNOWLEDGMENTS AND DISCLAIMERS

Credit for the fantastic cover design goes to Pamela Sinclair, *It Girl Designs*.

Thanks to my new editor, Martin O'Hearn. Your efforts make me look almost literate.

"Till the light dies in your eyes." Partial lyrics from Tarpon Jim, by Jim Morris.

The names of all participants except for Ed and Kim have been concealed for the author's legal protection.

The conclusions drawn and accusations made are strictly the editorial opinion of the author, and not proven facts.

ABOUT THE AUTHOR

Ed Robinson was a reporter and editor of a weekly newspaper, *The Smyrna Times*. He was also a contributing writer for *The Mariner Magazine*, a Maryland based publication covering all things boating and fishing. After twenty years working for a major utility, he quit his job and moved onto a boat. He and his wife Kim are somewhere on the west coast of Florida.

Contact Kim and Ed:
Kimandedrobinson@gmail.com
Join Ed on Facebook:
https://www.facebook.com/quityo
urjobandliveonaboat?ref=hl
Follow Ed's blog:
http://quityourjobandliveonaboat.wordpress.com/

OTHER BOOKS BY ED ROBINSON

LEAP OF FAITH: QUIT YOUR JOB AND LIVE ON A BOAT

There are many of us who dream about selling all our stuff, quitting our jobs, and running away to Paradise. This is a story about one couple who made that dream come true. The author shares what it feels like to experience ultimate freedom, and outlines the steps they took to get there. The story includes tales from their travels, social commentary on the state of today's American society, and a simple financial plan that will benefit anyone, regardless of their future goals. Throughout the narrative the reader is treated to dolphins and manatees, pelicans and osprey, blue skies, blue water and white sand beaches. Tropical music plays a role as well. Read how music inspired them to execute their plan. Follow along as they transform from everyday working drones to carefree boat bums and beachcombers. This book will make you rethink how you look at life, and money.

Amazon Bestseller for Happiness

POOP, BOOZE, AND BIKINIS

Ed Robinson's first book, *Leap of Faith: Quit Your Job and Live on a Boat*, was an Amazon best seller in multiple categories. Now he's back with this hilarious look at the nautical lifestyle. From Poop to Booze to Bikinis, he covers the funnier side of the issues encountered by boaters all of types. With chapters like Signs You Live on a Boat, Stupid People on Rental Equipment, and Zombies Can't Swim, you'll find plenty of laughs. There's even a chapter for Tim Dorsey fans. If you are a live-aboard, cruiser, weekender, wannabe boater, have boating friends, or are just a fan of Ed Robinson's wit, you will enjoy this light hearted romp through many maritime topics.

Amazon #1 Bestseller in Boating